Infertility

How Couples
Can Cope

Infertility

How Couples Can Cope

LINDA P. SALZER

G.K. HALL &CO.

70 LINCOLN STREET, BOSTON, MASS.

G. K. Hall & Co.
70 Lincoln Street
Boston, Massachusetts 02111

We wish to acknowledge the following sources for permission to reprint material in this book:

pp. 115–16: "Eliciting the Relaxation Response" from *The Relaxation Response* by Herbert Benson, M.D., with Miriam Z. Klipper. Copyright © 1975 by William Morrow and Company, Inc. Reprinted by permission of the publisher.

pp. 116–17: Dr. Edward Charlesworth and Ronald Nathan, excerpted from *Stress Management: A Comprehensive Guide to Wellness.* Copyright © 1984 by Edward A. Charlesworth, Ph.D., and Ronald G. Nathan, Ph.D. Reprinted with the permission of Atheneum Publishers, Inc.

pp. 249–50: "To an Adopted" by Carol Lynn Pearson from *The Search.* Copyright © 1970 by Carol Lynn Pearson. Reprinted by permission of Doubleday & Company, Inc.

Library of Congress Cataloging-in-Publication Data

Salzer, Linda P.
  Infertility: how couples can cope.

  Bibliography: p. 284
  Includes index.
  1. Infertility—Psychological aspects.
2. Adjustment (Psychology) I. Title.
RC889.S25 1986   616.6'92'0019   85-23654
ISBN 0-8161-8782-7
PB ISBN 0-8161-8798-3

Designed by Carole Rollins. Copyedited under the supervision of Michael Sims. Set in 10/13 ITC Garamond by R/TSI Typographic Co., Inc.

To our son, Eric—a dream come true.

Contents

Preface

"Do you have children?" Such an ordinary question—but for the couple facing infertility, it brings thoughts of temperature charts, doctors' appointments, marital conflict, and sex on schedule. The struggle to have a child can turn your life on end and change a calm, well-adjusted person into a bundle of nerves. I know—I've been there.

My husband and I struggled with infertility for many years. Although the intense pain has lessened since the joyous arrival of our adopted son, the memories of that struggle remain as vivid as if they occurred yesterday. How do you forget the awkward dinner party where everyone else is proudly displaying pictures of their children? Or the daily awakening to thermometer and Pergonal injections? Or the frustration and fatigue from month after month of doctors' appointments? Then just when you think there might be an answer to your problems, new difficulties and disappointments arise. We were very fortunate to have the wonderful support of family, friends, and the infertility organization, RESOLVE, but even with all this help, we found the experience of infertility to be devastating.

Although I had been trained professionally to deal with life crises, nothing had prepared me for the impact of being infertile. When we were first told of our problems, I immediately read everything I could lay my hands on. I approached the situation intellectually, methodically—just as I'd always tackled a new problem. But, although I became very knowledgeable about the medical aspects of infertility, there was no book to turn to for handling the emotional upheaval. My husband and I couldn't talk to each other and I was sure no one else could understand. I would break into tears at the sight of a pregnant woman or a baby carriage. I questioned myself and my life, searching for an answer to what was happening.

Remembering my own dark days, I wanted to write this book especially for those people who are overwhelmed by feelings of despair and are afraid they will never hold a baby in their arms, and for those who feel isolated and are struggling to relate to a fertile world that seems to have left them behind. Remember this: you are not alone. There are at least 10 million others who are dealing with this crisis, which means one out of every six couples of childbearing age.

But infertility today carries great promise as well as misery. As medical science progresses and infertile couples turn in desperation to the newest techniques, they learn there is hope for many of them—reproductive knowledge and technology are skyrocketing! It is now estimated that 60 to 70 percent of all infertile couples can be successfully treated. But, even as the media extol the triumphs of these new procedures, the day-to-day emotional strain is too often ignored. Those who have become involved in in vitro fertilization or surrogate parenting understand very well the emotional toll exacted by their efforts to conceive.

If you have been diagnosed as infertile, you are probably living in a no-man's-land where time is marked only by the day of your cycle and the treatment you are currently undergoing. Emotions run rampant and you may often question whether you and your marriage can survive. Chances are that you are terrified by the unknown: perhaps you are facing a medical crisis for the first time in your life, not knowing what the future will hold and feeling emotionally out of control. This book aims to help you understand the myriad of feelings you will experience during infertility and to recognize that these feelings are normal. It will also provide you with some ways of coping that many have found to be effective. For example, how do you endure holidays when family togetherness is emphasized and you are supposed to be feeling happy? What do you do when every friend and relative seem magically to be getting pregnant? How do you keep your marriage from dissolving when communication has become nonexistent and sex unfulfilling? Your struggle with infertility can affect all areas of your life—social and family relationships, marriage, employment, physical health, religious faith, and personal growth. This book explores all these areas and illustrates them with firsthand experiences. These personal accounts are sensitively shared by people who *know* what it's like to be infertile. Although the book won't solve your medical problems, it will help you keep

your marriage strong, find support from others, and maintain a positive self-image.

Remember that this is a book for both men and women because
infertility physically and emotionally affects both sexes. Each of you
needs to face and work through your feelings before you can come
to terms with the situation as a couple. But what do you do if your
spouse refuses to talk or the two of you can't agree on a course of
treatment? The emphasis in this book is on open communication
between partners.

Most important, I hope to show you that there *can* be an end to
the pain of infertility, although each couple's resolution may differ.
This book helps you recognize when it's time to stop the heroics of
treatment and whether you are stuck. It shows you how to define
your needs as an individual and couple so you can choose wisely
among the available options—adoption, childfree living, or alternative means of having biological children. For example, is your primary goal that of being a parent or is it the pregnancy and birth
experience you do not want to miss? In my own life, I had never
thought that adoption would be our answer, but it was. It provided a
wonderful sense of peace at the close of an exceedingly difficult
time for us.

As you read, remember that the stage you are at—first recognizing your infertility, being knee-deep in treatment, learning to accept
the situation, or coming to terms with it—will affect how you are
presently reacting to the crisis. The particular causes of your infertility and whether or not a diagnosis can be made may also have a
strong influence. Those, for example, with "unexplained infertility"
seem to experience greater difficulty in calling an end to their
medical efforts than do those with a clear-cut diagnosis. In addition,
the issue of which of you has the medical problem will influence
your feelings. Although infertility always affects both partners, guilt
or blame may be particularly troublesome when only one of you has
a difficulty.

You might want to read through this book from beginning to
end or you might prefer to dip into it from time to time as specific
issues arise. Remember, though, that this book is intended to help
prevent problems, as well as to deal with them once they exist. Even
though a particular subject, such as doctor-patient communication,
may not be a problem for you now, reading through that chapter can
help you avoid future difficulties. Remember, too, that there are no

absolutes when it comes to infertility. Although people share many common responses to the crisis, they react to it in their own personal ways. By reading the examples here, you may derive your own effective way for handling infertility.

You will find that a variety of options are discussed here that you may not want to consider now but that may be useful in the future. Whatever you decide, the critical point is that you regain control of yourself and resume living. The answers are not simple, nor do they come quickly; but I hope that in reading and using this book you will find it is possible to survive this life-shattering event—with happiness and fulfillment.

Acknowledgments

Conceiving and giving birth to this book has been part of my own resolution to infertility. It began as a good project to work on at home but quickly became an endeavor of the heart, both rewarding and emotionally draining. It is something I would never have accomplished without the help and support of many relatives, friends, and others.

First, I thank my husband, Rick, who encouraged my outlandish fantasy of writing a book and stood by me during the early frustrations of learning about the publishing business. For two years, he was willing to give up our kitchen table to a computer, piles of books, and endless notes, never complaining when the book took precedence over having a clean house. I also thank my wonderful son, Eric, who brought such joy to my life that it inspired me to write about the resolution of infertility. He miraculously continued to take two-hour naps every afternoon, thus giving me an opportunity to write.

Along the way, the interest and support from my family (both my own and my husband's), as well as many friends, have meant a great deal. They stood by me not only during the writing of this book but also during the many earlier years of infertility tests and treatment.

Many of the sensitive experiences and feelings described in this book are the anonymous contributions of RESOLVE members from throughout the United States. I sincerely thank them for their help in this endeavor.

The staff of the Englewood Hospital Library was very helpful in gathering journal articles from libraries throughout the area. Many organizations also took the time to send brochures, articles, and newsletters. These include the Endometriosis Association; Latin

America Parents Association; Stepping Stones; the Open Door Society of Massachusetts, Inc.; Families Adopting Children Everywhere; National Committee for Adoption; Ours, Inc.; Parents for Private Adoption; Infertility Center of New York; Surrogate Mothering, Ltd.; Hagar Institute; and William W. Handel.

I am especially indebted to Beverly Freeman, director of RE-SOLVE, INC., for her enthusiastic interest in my book. She not only helped in my search for a publisher but also carefully reviewed my manuscript.

Finally, I give very special thanks to my editor, Janice Meagher, who patiently led me through each step and always had an encouraging word. She made the experience far more enjoyable than I ever imagined. I thank her not only for her skill as an editor but, even more important, her warmth and sensitivity.

Infertility:
The Silent Struggle

What Is Infertility?

Infertility does not kill, nor is it a visible disorder. It is rarely discussed in public and its sufferers usually do not receive flowers or condolences. It is a private experience revealed only by one's childlessness and on occasion perhaps a few uncontrolled tears. No wonder so few people understand the impact of this devastating and growing problem.

Infertility may be defined as the inability to become pregnant after one year of having regular sexual relations without use of contraception, or as the inability to conceive and carry a baby to live birth. Since it is the woman who becomes pregnant and delivers a baby, often she is thought to be the only "culprit" in infertility, but that is not so. Female factors and male factors each account for about 35 percent of the problems in infertility cases. Not uncommonly, both partners have a reproductive difficulty, the situation in 20 percent of the cases. In the remaining 10 percent of cases doctors are unable to identify any medical reason for the problem.[1] Because men and women share equally in this condition, *both* partners always must be thoroughly evaluated.

What Goes Wrong?

The act of conception is an intricate and fragile course of events. First there is the manufacture of sperm, which must travel through a microscopic tunnel that twists and turns on the way to a storage area. There they remain until ejaculation occurs. Although a tremendous number of sperm (normally anywhere from 40 to 150 million) are released during a single ejaculation, less than 10 percent will survive the hostile environment of the vagina.[2] Then follows the journey through the cervix and uterus to the fallopian tubes, a precarious trek that less than a hundred sperm will accomplish. Of those, some will enter the wrong tube, while others will become entrapped in the irregularities of the passageway. To further inhibit this journey, the remaining sperm must travel against the current to encounter an egg.

Meanwhile, countless other factors in the woman are determining the production and release of the one egg that normally matures each month. The menstrual cycle is a complex hormonal process that allows for the development of eggs, the preparation of the cervix to allow sperm to enter, and the changes in the uterus that make it receptive to a fertilized egg. Conception, then, is the result of a miraculous and complex system—so complex it is amazing that conception ever takes place at all.

Given this complexity, it is easy to understand the great potential for the system to go wrong. It also means that dozens of difficulties are included under the umbrella of infertility. In the woman, causes of infertility can include endocrine disorders that interfere with ovulation, endometriosis (a condition in which part of the endometrium, or lining of the uterus, is found outside the uterus), pelvic infections, structural abnormalities of the uterus, and cervical problems. The majority of female infertility problems are the result of pelvic infections, which can damage and block the fallopian tubes.[3] Tubal blockage can also be caused by endometriosis, which many professionals believe is on the increase. About one-fourth to one-third of all female infertility problems are now linked to this condition.[4] Endometriosis has mistakenly been nicknamed "the career woman's disease." Although there may be a relationship between delayed childbirth and the occurrence of endometriosis, this disease frequently develops during adolescence, often going undiagnosed. Endometriosis can also appear or reappear in women who have previously been pregnant. Unfortunately, the causes are not known. Ovulation impairments (failure to ovulate or erratic ovulation) are responsible for around 20 percent of all female problems.[5]

Causes of male infertility are also diverse. They may involve a varicocele (varicose veins in the scrotum), testicular failure, infection in the reproductive tract, hormonal imbalances, use of certain drugs, adult mumps, retrograde ejaculation, or injury to the reproductive organs. Any of these may lead to problems with sperm production (inadequate numbers, poor motility, abnormal structure), but about 30 percent of cases involving low sperm count are caused by a varicocele.[6]

Problems do not have to be major, however, to cause infertility. Even slight difficulties, especially if experienced by both partners, can interfere with conception.

When Should You Get Help?

Although couples are considered infertile after one year of unsuccessful efforts to conceive, the emotional elements of the problem can involve other time scales. Couples may become concerned about reproductive failure at varying points. One couple, for example, may desire a child but be in no particular hurry; they will wait then for several years before making medical inquiries. But others may become anxious after six months and quickly pursue medical intervention. There is no *right* time to become worried, but it should be remembered that, even among the most fertile population (women in their early twenties), studies have shown that the average time to conceive is four to five months.

On the other hand, many people do have a legitimate basis for inquiring about an infertility problem early in their efforts, perhaps after six months. Women over the age of thirty have reason to be concerned not only because their fertility is declining (the "biological clock") but also because risks of an abnormal pregnancy begin to increase at this age. In addition, individuals who have experienced any problem in the past that might impair fertility should certainly begin questioning at an early point: a man who has had adult mumps with inflammation of the testes or who was born with undescended testicles, or a woman with a history of an irregular menstrual cycle, endometriosis, or cessation of her period.

Thus, differences in couples' ages, histories, and perceptions must be taken into account. A general guideline might be that you would be wise to contact an infertility specialist either after one year of unsuccessful effort or at the point when anxiety is adversely affecting you or your relationship with your spouse.

Who Is Infertile?

Infertility knows no boundaries. It afflicts people of all races, of all economic classes, and in all geographic areas. Over the past twenty years, the incidence of infertility has almost tripled, yet few people are aware of the magnitude of the problem.[7] Approximately 10 million people in the United States experience infertility, which means one out of every five couples of childbearing age. Although you may feel you're the only one with this problem, the chances are you have neighbors, friends, or colleagues who are experiencing the same difficulty.

Although the peak fertility time for women is between the ages of 18 and 25 and the ability to reproduce lessens after that, decisions to begin a family increasingly are being postponed to well past these years. Maturity and marital stability are two advantages of raising children at a later age, but the flip side of waiting is the loss of fertility. Delayed conception itself has contributed significantly to the increased infertility rate, as has the greater possibility of developing endometriosis as one grows older.

But there has been in recent years an enormous rise in the occurrence of infertility among younger adults, too. The rate jumped 177 percent from 1965 to 1982 among married women aged twenty to twenty-four.[8] There are several explanations for the increase. People are becoming sexually active at an earlier age, making it more likely that a person will have multiple partners during premarital years and increasing the possibility of contracting venereal disease, a common cause of infertility. Abortion also has been on the rise and with it comes some risk of infection (low estimates range from 1 to 5 percent).[9] Birth control methods, too, are more widely used, and at least one form, the IUD, has been shown to lead to pelvic inflammatory disease, an infection of the uterus and fallopian tubes.

Prenatal exposure to DES (diethylstilbestrol, a drug that was once prescribed to pregnant women to increase chances for a successful pregnancy) may also be an important factor for both men and women now of reproductive age. One result of DES in women has been structural abnormalities of the reproductive system, causing repeated miscarriages.

Among males, it has been shown that sperm counts have markedly decreased across all age brackets, possibly because of environmental pollution or stress.[10] Much less is known about male infertility, however, since the focus of research has primarily been on women. Studies on the causes of impaired sperm production are long overdue.

Correcting Some Misconceptions about Infertility

Inaccurate ideas about infertility are rampant among the lay public. The following are a few of the striking misconceptions held by too many people:

1. Infertility indicates a sexual dysfunction.
   Fact: There is usually no causal relationship between sexual performance and the ability to conceive.

2. Being infertile means that you must have a lot of fun trying to conceive.
   Fact: This is far from true. Sex on schedule is rarely fun; in fact, sexual relationships often deteriorate as a result of infertility.

3. Infertility is a woman's problem.
   Fact: Men experience infertility with the same frequency as do women. Both men and women need to be carefully evaluated when problems develop in trying to conceive.

4. Being able to get pregnant once means that you will never experience infertility at a later point in life.
   Fact: Secondary infertility, defined as the inability to successfully give birth again after having delivered one child, is a common phenomenon. One study has indicated that secondary infertility afflicts approximately 60 percent of couples having problems conceiving.[11]

5. Infertility is caused by psychological problems.
   Fact: In about 90 percent of all cases, a physical condition can be identified as causing the infertility. Infertility *leads* to stress and emotional difficulties; it has not been proved to be the result of them.

6. Adoption is a means of ensuring a later pregnancy.
   Fact: The rate at which adoptive parents spontaneously

conceive is about the same as for couples who have not adopted. Pregnancy after adoption occurs in only 5 percent of cases.

7. Seeking medical help for this problem is fruitless.
Fact: It is estimated that 70 percent of infertile couples can be helped to produce biological children.[12]

The Medical Scene Today

Medical science is advancing in this area as in others. Problems that just a few years ago were without solution can now often be treated. Only 40 percent of all infertility cases could be diagnosed ten years ago, compared to 90 percent today.[13] Better diagnostic procedures and a variety of new treatments have brought promise to what in the past was a pessimistic outlook for infertile couples. The number of medical specialists in this field has also increased enormously. Specialists can now be found in many areas of medicine, including urology (in the subspecialty of andrology), gynecology, and endocrinology have increased, too.

In some ways, however, these advances have been a mixed blessing. Although many have been helped, false hopes have been raised that *all* infertility problems can be successfully treated. For those who have undergone long drawn-out treatments because there always seemed to be some new procedure to investigate, it can be very difficult to reach resolution by some other means, such as AID, adoption, or childfree living.

The Crisis of Infertility

Most people assume that fertility is a God-given and biological right, a certainty that will occur at a planned moment in their lives. They assume that starting a family will be a decision they control, like pursuing a career, getting married, or selecting friends. Many for years have used birth control devices that have been perfected to almost 100 percent reliability.

When I think back to all those years on the pill and using an IUD, I'm not sure whether to laugh or cry. It now seems ludicrous that I worried so much over the possibility of an unplanned pregnancy. In those days,

*the first glimpse of my period was often a relief, a
confirmation that my life was proceeding as planned.
How different from the feeling I have today!*

Discovering that you are infertile is more than just another
stressful event in your life. It is a developmental crisis that holds
significant meaning and far-reaching consequences for the people it
affects. Often, it is the first crisis of a person's life and probably the
first intensive contact with the medical profession.

*I've been infertile for four years and have been through
three surgeries, countless doctors' appointments, and a
myriad of drugs. The effects on my life and my
marriage have been enormous. In some respects, I feel
that my life has just come to a standstill. It's been,
without doubt, the toughest experience I've ever faced.*

A crisis occurs whenever you face a difficulty that you are
unable to solve with your customary coping skills. You become
disorganized and confused, often making many unsuccessful efforts
at solving the problem. Being confronted by failure and helplessness,
you feel increasingly anxious and immobilized. This is what happens
when you are faced with infertility.

How people respond to a crisis, however, varies significantly.
Some are able to resume their normal level of functioning when the
crisis ends, but others find their ability to function declining or
strengthening. It is in any case a turning point. The fact that previous
coping mechanisms may be only partially successful for managing a
new crisis implies that in crises there is not only an opportunity for
significant growth, as new ways of coping are developed, but also the
chance of deterioration.

*Trying to cope with infertility has been very difficult. It
feels similar to living with a chronic illness—it's always
there. Before I discovered my infertility problem, a series
of family tragedies occurred. I learned coping skills and
worked through all the pain, only to discover that none
seemed to work with the crisis of infertility.*

The unusual feature about infertility is that it is usually composed of a series of crises—which means never-ending stress. Each month brings the anxiety of new tests and treatments, not to mention the repeated disappointment when menstruation occurs. To complicate matters, you and your partner will probably experience the crisis differently.

Infertility is called a developmental crisis because it directly influences a person's ability to master effectively the growth tasks of early adulthood. Raising children is seen by most as a principal goal of adult life, and infertility poses a threat to its accomplishment. Erik Erikson, the theorist of ego psychology, developed a sequence of eight psychosocial stages a person experiences during a lifetime. The tasks of each must be successfully completed in order to achieve success in later stages.

He describes the stage of *generativity* as "primarily the concern of establishing and guiding the next generation." He adds that "mature man needs to be needed, and maturity needs guidance as well as encouragement from what has been produced and must be taken care of."[14] Generativity refers to all kinds of creative, productive, nurturing behavior, such as artistic accomplishments, community work, or teaching, so that being childless does not necessarily mean that you will fail at this task. But, if you cannot produce children, and you neglect the alternatives, your childlessness could become a major block in the successful resolution of this stage. The result may be what Erikson calls stagnation and personal impoverishment.

Such failure would affect a person's management of the eighth and final stage of development, *ego integrity*. Mastering this last stage means arriving at the point where you are at peace with yourself and your life. Erikson states that failure to do so will result in a sense of despair and a fear of death. It is the pain of feeling alone, dissatisfied, and unproductive.

Coming Out of the Closet

One of the most painful aspects of infertility is this sense of being alone. Isolation develops easily because the infertile person tends to say very little about the problem to anyone and is very sensitive to others' comments about having children. It is often kept a secret between partners, shared only with family and close friends if even those people can be trusted. The fear of being pitied or looked down upon is often intense. However, the pressure of enduring the situation alone can be equally, if not more, distressing.

Deciding to share your dilemma with another person is a difficult milestone in the process of learning to live with infertility, but it is well worth the risk. And often the fear of taking this step is worse than actually doing so. Many find that a tremendous burden is lifted when they are able to tell another person, without embarrassment, that they cannot have children. Infertility is a personal matter, certainly, and does not have to be announced to everyone, but telling a few select people may help immensely.

There are, of course, risks in opening up to others. Certainly, some people will not understand or will make insensitive remarks. As Erma Bombeck once said in a column on the topic, there are times when infertile people "get about as much sympathy as an 83-pound woman trying to gain weight."[15] There will also be times of uncomfortable silence when you regret having brought up the subject. But the potential gain in support and understanding from opening that door can be immeasurable.

Society too needs to be educated, and silence only perpetuates ignorance. Accepting and acknowledging infertility is a difficult step but one that eventually must be taken. As Bombeck wrote, "Closets are without air. They cannot sustain life."[16]

The Emotional
Roller Coaster

*I cannot conceive or bear children; I am infertile. My
infertility is a blow to my self-esteem, a violation of
my privacy, an assault on my sexuality, a final exam
on my ability to cope, an affront to my sense of justice,
a painful reminder that nothing can be taken for
granted. My infertility is a break in the continuity of
life. It is, above all, a wound—to my body, to my
psyche, to my soul. The pain is intense.*[1]

Ask anyone who has been through infertility and he or she will
probably tell you the same thing—"It was like nothing I've ever
been through before." Infertility is powerful and often destructive,
dredging up emotions that you may never have known were inside
you. It catapults you from the heights of hope to the depths of
despair, all in a moment's time. The analogy to a roller-coaster ride is
apt, except that there often appears to be no end in sight.

Barbara Eck Menning, the founder of RESOLVE, first suggested
that the psychological stages experienced in mourning might be
applicable to the upheaval felt in infertility. Clearly, many of the
feelings are similar—anger, guilt, depression—all part of accepting
the loss. But there is a major difference. Reaching a point of resolution with infertility, accepting it, is usually a very long time in
coming.

You have probably all experienced some type of loss in your
life—death of a loved one, loss of a job, divorce—but infertility is
different. It is an intangible loss that catches you unprepared for its
impact. You can't quite grab hold of it, and yet the pain is very real.

10

To make matters worse, few people without firsthand experience have much understanding of what it is like.

Searching for an answer takes over your life. Because the medical findings are confusing and the solutions varied, the search can go on and on. Maybe next month a baby will come—with the next test, the next treatment, the next doctor.

In this chapter I will describe the normal emotional responses to infertility and why it can be so debilitating. I hope that those of you who are infertile will see yourselves in these pages and recognize that what is happening to you is normal, not "crazy."

Childhood Fantasies and Expectations

So much in our lives is taken for granted—having good health, being able to see and hear and walk freely, having caring people around. Certainly one of our assumptions is that we will be able to bear children. Most of us just take it for granted that someday we will become parents. We may consider postponing this role because of other important commitments in our lives, or we may even question the role itself—whether it is right for us. But, chances are, we have never given any serious thought to *not being able* to have children.

The seeds for this belief in becoming a parent are sown early in childhood. Children identify with significant adults in their lives, especially their parents. They play house and act out the roles of mother and father, mimicking the behaviors they observe in their homes. They watch other adults around them—grandparents, neighbors—again incorporating their perceptions of these people as "parents." The old childhood rhyme of "First comes love, then comes marriage, then comes _____ with a baby carriage!" is innocently chanted. The seven-year-old informs her parents how many children she expects to have, including the number of boys and girls. This has already been given careful consideration. Although as children grow older, they begin to appreciate that the adults in their lives play many roles, it is the role of parent that is understood earliest.

During adolescence and early adulthood, other developmental issues take precedence over that of becoming a parent, but the dream of having children does not disappear—instead, it is just put on a back burner. Although some of you may have experienced early indications of a reproductive problem and thus were suspicious about what the future might bring, it is likely that most of you never considered the possibility of infertility.

> *Not in my wildest dreams did I ever imagine I'd be infertile. I just assumed I'd become a mother like everyone else. From my earliest days playing with dolls to my teenage years as a babysitter and into early adulthood as a teacher, there was never any question of bearing a child. The thought was never "if"; it was "when."*

Even if you knew a childless couple or a family with adopted children, infertility was probably viewed as something that happens to others, not to *you*.

Many young adults are interested at first only in how to avoid the predicament of unexpected conception. With the media sounding warnings about the population explosion and parents issuing commands to be careful, who would think that someday there might be the opposite problem? It is no wonder that our early experiences are the roots of the intense emotions we later feel in response to infertility.

Emotional Stages of Infertility

An array of feelings appears during the infertility experience. In fact, it may be the first time you have been subjected to such an explosion of emotions—anger, guilt, fear, sadness, shame. When and how these feelings occur will differ from person to person, but usually they will be present at some point as you work toward resolution of the crisis. I have divided this process into four stages: (1) shock and denial ("Not me"), (2) responding to the assault ("Why me?" and "What can we do?"), (3) grieving ("Letting go"), and (4) acceptance ("Enough is enough" and "It's time to move on"). Although I have presented these stages as a progression, the response to infertility does not necessarily occur in such a structured, straightforward manner. Coping with infertility is full of twists and turns, with progress and setbacks. Nor are the stages mutually exclusive. Nevertheless, this list indicates a general course of emotional response.

It should be remembered, too, that the process can easily repeat itself. That is one of the unfortunate aspects of experiencing infertility.

> *When my husband was first tested, we learned of his very low sperm count and went through all the trauma created by this blow. After unsuccessful surgery, we cried together and spent considerable time soul-searching before we came to the conclusion that* AID *[donor insemination] was our only answer. Meanwhile, I had been tested and, although a few problems were indicated, I seemed capable of conceiving. We spent the next year using* AID *but to no avail. By that time, more extensive testing was necessary for me and it became clear that my tubes, partially open the year before, were now totally blocked. The emotional shock, the treatments, and the grieving process began all over again.*

Because your problem involves two people and because treating infertility is still an inexact science, an experience like this is not unlikely. Crises can occur over and over again.

Shock and Denial

> *"Not me."*

> *"I don't believe this is true."*

> *"That doctor is crazy—he doesn't know what he's talking about. We'll speak to someone else."*

> *"It can't be happening to us."*

After years, probably, of birth control and the confident assumption that children are an important part of our future, it is a cruel awakening to suddenly find that conception may not come easily or perhaps at all. Most of us have been relatively healthy throughout our lives and have spent little time in doctors' offices. Then suddenly we are struck with the news that something in our body is "wrong."

> *At first, the simple tests indicated a slight cervical mucous problem that didn't bother me too much. My*

husband's sperm count was fine, so I wasn't thinking of
any major problems. Then I had a hysterosalpingogram
which showed major blockage of the left tube and total
obstruction of the right one. My reaction—total
disbelief! I had absolutely no idea that things were this
bad. Never in a million years would I have thought this
could happen.

Many feel "stupid" that they struggled so long to avoid pregnancy
and now learn that they probably could not have conceived without
medical intervention anyway. Although this is a common reaction, it
must be remembered that a person's fertility can change as years
pass. Those with secondary infertility can easily attest to that.

Denial or disbelief is likely when the news of infertility is sudden and unexpected. Those who become aware of infertility gradually or who are tested with only vague results may never respond
this way. But denial, when it does occur, is a defense mechanism that
serves an important function. It screens the person from the initial
devastating pain and provides time to assimilate what has
happened—like a temporary anesthesia.

I hurt so much that the only way I could deal with it
was through denial. I didn't tell anyone and my
husband and I rarely discussed it. When we did, I
always ended up crying and feeling as if I was losing
my mind. At that time, there was no definitive
diagnosis, so I continued to ignore the problem and
hope.

I suppose I "learned" of my infertility problem nearly
five years before it really sunk in. That's how much
time had elapsed between the point I was told no
sperm were found in a specimen and the day I
underwent surgery. Only when I was told, after the
operation, that my problem could not be surgically
repaired did I really accept the extent of the infertility.
It was only then that I felt depressed, confused, and
somewhat guilty about my inability to be a father.

Denial becomes problematic or unhealthy only when it goes on for too long a time, so that the individual does not adjust to reality. People who refuse to seek medical treatment or who turn a deaf ear to unequivocal medical findings fall into this category. These people simply avoid the issue or rationalize ("I've just been working too hard"). Another form of denial is to place the blame on the spouse, refusing to accept any responsibility for dealing with the problem. Others totally relinquish responsibility, pretending that the doctor or God or someone must "take over" because they are incapable of handling it. Although infertility certainly promotes out-of-control feelings, it is important to remember that there are things you can and must do if you want to have a child.

Long-term denial may be especially problematic if one spouse perceives the situation realistically and the other is stuck in denial. In such cases, it is important for the "realistic" partner to recognize what is happening and to obtain the help of a third party, perhaps the doctor or a counselor, who can assist the couple. Rather than trying to batter away at the denial, which can be frustrating and ineffective, it is necessary to understand its purpose. The painful and frightening feelings it masks need to be explored.

Some people suspect, long before a definitive diagnosis is made, that they are going to have a problem. In these cases, the phase of shock and denial may never exist, although chances are that some denial has occurred along the way.

> *I wasn't at all surprised to learn of my infertility. I had always suspected I would have a problem because my periods were very irregular. To compound this, I was very ambivalent about pregnancy, motherhood, and femininity, so I viewed my infertility as something to be expected. I guess I assumed, though, that if I really made a decision to be a mother, the difficulty might go away.*

> *I always knew I had a problem. While my girlfriends were having abortions, I was "proud" that I was so careful. But when I met my future husband and we were having unprotected intercourse for two years, I knew there was a problem for sure. It was only after a year of marriage that I went to a gynecologist to inquire what might be wrong. When he signed my*

insurance form diagnosis as "infertility," I cried all the
way home—the truth was now in black and white. My
intuition was painfully correct.

Responding to the Assault

The second stage is characterized by an obsession with trying to
determine what has happened, what you have done wrong, why you
are being put through this agony when everyone else can conceive
so easily. During this time, there is also an intense focus on the
multitude of infertility tests and treatments. This may be a very long
phase of the infertility process.

Enduring the actual treatments has been the most
stressful part of infertility for me. It begins with
collecting urine samples from cycle day 8 to day 14 to
look for LH surge. The samples must be brought in on
specific days, with a one-and-a-half-hour trip each way.
Then, whenever, the urine shows the surge, I have to get
a sperm sample from my husband, rush to the doctor's
office, and hope and pray that the intrauterine
insemination won't be painful (it usually is). Then I
lay there on the table alone, staring at a white ceiling
for a half hour. It is only when I leave, and the cycle
monitoring is over, that I feel a great sense of relief and
wonder whether I can go through another month like
this.

The actual responses displayed will be unique to each individual, reflecting earlier behavior patterns. Early emotional conflicts and
unresolved losses will tend to reappear at this time of crisis, often
with renewed pain. How you react to infertility will follow the
manner in which you have handled other crises in your life. For
example, if you are a fighter and have a positive attitude toward life,
you will probably approach the problem of infertility in a similar
style. But if you tend to become overwhelmed, viewing yourself and
your life pessimistically, your response will probably be no different
now. Try to be aware of your own approach and consider whether it
is a help or a hindrance. Recognize too that many intense feelings

are likely to surface during this stage, including anger, guilt, depression, and a sense of isolation.

ANGER

Anger results from your feelings of vulnerability and helplessness; you lack control over your body, your emotions, your future. Until now, you have had a sense of command over your life: you chose your mate, decided where to live, picked a career, selected friends. What a blow to find that something else you felt was a matter of choice has been decided for you! It is inevitable that you should feel angry at everything and everybody around you—especially at the unfairness of life.

> *I always considered myself to be an exceptionally strong, "together" person. In my life, I had weathered other crises and come out unscathed. But, all of a sudden, I was struck with a situation that I didn't seem to be able to handle. It was like being hurled around in a cyclone, completely helpless—sobbing, horrible anxiety, and night after night of sleeplessness. I finally realized that this was the first time in my life when I faced a problem that no matter how hard I tried I couldn't solve. My usual coping skill of "taking the bull by the horns" and putting all my effort into getting what I wanted suddenly didn't work. I was frightened and angry at my inability to do anything.*

How you handle your anger has important ramifications. Becoming angry at yourself is likely to lead to depression; being angry at others only upsets them and may set up walls between you so they cannot help. Anger is often vented at friends who seem to conceive so easily and do not have to deal with this disruption in their lives.

> *Anger at and jealousy of other fertile people have been overwhelming for me. I resent their success and happiness. I hate this emotion but feel unable to control it. One of the most sickening feelings I have had during my six years of infertility is like no other I have ever had. In learning of another's pregnancy, I am*

> *physically shaken and then go into a sobbing*
> *depression, sometimes lasting a few hours. I feel*
> *physically ill at another's good fortune—it is dreadful!*
> *I then feel guilty that I can no longer feel happiness for*
> *others on the occasion of their pregnancy or childbirth.*
> *Sometimes, when someone has a miscarriage, I don't*
> *even feel sorry for them. Then I feel ashamed.*

Anger may be aimed at spouses for causing the infertility problem, for not understanding, or for not making more of an effort. Blaming your partner can be one of the most destructive behaviors at this time. Also common is projecting anger upon individuals or establishments who have some degree of control over you, especially physicians or adoption agencies. The actual target of your anger, however, is often yourself and your unhappy situation. But because being furious at yourself may be too painful and the situation too diffuse, it is easier to project these feelings upon others.

> *I want to be angry at somebody, but who? I can't*
> *blame the doctor—he's telling us the truth. I can't*
> *blame my spouse—he hasn't done this on purpose.*
> *Somehow being angry at God seems sinful. I don't feel*
> *this anger daily, but when I do I take it out on other*
> *people and situations by overreacting.*

Still another target for anger may be the unborn child. Some couples may begin to question if a baby is worth all this painful effort; if a child could make up for all the grief it's "causing."

Anger is directed most effectively at the circumstances of infertility—at having to receive daily injections or needing to turn your life upside down for frequent medical appointments. This is a direct and reasonable target. Then sharing this anger with your spouse or a close friend, putting it into writing, or engaging in physical activity to release the tension and rage can be cathartic. When sharing it with another person, though, make it clear that you just need to ventilate, that you're not angry with them. Although it may seem that there are only two ways of handling your fury—taking it out on somebody else or keeping it bottled up inside—it is possible to express your anger in a constructive way by sharing your reasons for it. And feel reassured that your feelings of outrage over the unfairness of the situation are legitimate.

Anger, however, may also become more irrational—you may strongly resent anyone with a large family or express your anger in a manner that is out of proportion to what triggered it. Irrational feelings like these are often a disguise for an intense anger the person is afraid to express directly. Try to recognize when your rage is destroying yourself or your relationships with others because it is being vented in the wrong direction.

Although anger is a natural and normal response to infertility, there will be those of you who are frightened by this feeling and find it difficult to express. This discomfort may be the result of rigid religious training that condemned any expression of rage. Or anger may be associated in your mind with disastrous outcomes, such as severe punishment, abandonment, or destructive behavior. So you may deny ("I don't feel angry—after all, we have each other"), intellectualize ("There's no reason for me to be angry"), or rationalize ("Things could always be worse") your feelings of rage. The trouble with these approaches is that you may fail to acknowledge your real feelings and thus never deal with them effectively. The anger, then, is likely to surface elsewhere, which will take its toll. Self-destructive behaviors are often the result of unresolved anger.

When a feeling of being out of control emerges, a grasping at magic and superstition sometimes appears, even among the most sophisticated people.

> *I'm almost embarrassed to admit it, but I found myself with a stash of good luck charms during my infertility—several four-leaf clovers, a white elephant necklace, a red ribbon tied to my bed, a positive horoscope, and a fortune from a Chinese fortune cookie that said my dreams would come true! Clearly, my medical efforts weren't getting me anywhere, so I had to put my faith in something else. I felt so angry and out of control that I needed to feel there was something that would make a difference.*

You'd be surprised how many people dealing with the problem of infertility resort to these beliefs!

The anger will eventually subside if you express it and work it through. Support groups can be very helpful in this regard; becoming well informed also can be useful. By learning about your situation and establishing some control over your treatment, you combat your feeling of helplessness. This may be threatening to some physicians, but those experienced in treating infertility problems will understand the importance of your need.

GUILT

Guilt is another common response during the assault phase. You may wonder why this feeling is so strong now. It reflects the fact that most of us need to perceive the world as a sensible, orderly place in which cause-effect relationships exist. We want to believe there is a reason for everything that happens. We search, then, for some explanation of our infertility, and often the cause we focus on is some behavior in our past we feel guilty about. This may be premarital or extramarital sex, venereal disease, use of birth control, incestuous thoughts, promiscuity, masturbation, abortion, or homosexual fantasies and experiences. Infertility thus becomes the "punishment."

> *Infertility has made me feel so old. I now look "back" and see all the mistakes I've made that probably have led to the infertility. I get angry when my period comes and feel guilty because of my promiscuous past. I see that part of my life and the image of myself as very negative. Infertility has made me feel my mortality, and makes me even more anxious to have a baby, to present that part of me and the one I love to the world. My self-esteem has never been the greatest, and infertility definitely hasn't helped.*

> *I am a conscientious, hardworking, achievement-oriented person and don't like being helpless, not in control of a goal I want and need very badly. Sometimes I think God is punishing me for the abortion I had 4 1/2 years ago. If only I could relive that time.*

People can be harsh with themselves. In their search to find an answer, they play judge and jury with their own lives, condemning themselves for all-too-human errors ("At 17, I got pregnant and had an abortion—now I'm paying for it") or expecting themselves to have foreseen the future ("If only we'd had children when we were younger. I now feel I was selfish in wanting to establish a career"). Self-blame like this can result from our feeling that we should be perfect. The reality, however, is that no one is perfect. We all make mistakes, and none of us can predict what the future holds.

Particularly susceptible to blaming themselves for their infertility are people who grew up in an atmosphere of criticism. Either they always found fault with themselves or others dwelt on their shortcomings. Some people too experience a vague sense of guilt without recognizing any event that precipitated it. As one woman said, "I feel like I have received a sentence for some kind of moral crime. I know it's irrational, but I can't help wondering what I did to deserve this."

Guilt may also result from the demands of treatment and your resentment of them—the pressure of feeling that you must do everything you can to conceive.

Guilt has been very difficult for me to handle. The infertility problem is mine—as far as who needs surgery. My husband says it's my decision because I'm the one who will have to endure another major operation. He doesn't want to force me into it. But I have feelings of guilt that if I don't go ahead, I'm denying him his chance to have a natural child. How could I do that to him?

The guilt-anger combination has caused me to live in anguish. Long-distance running has long been one of my most pleasurable activities, and yet I always suspected (and the endocrinologists have confirmed) that this is contributing to my infertility. I feel I have to limit it and that makes me very angry—angry at the situation for being so unfair and angry at myself for my inability to change. Whenever I run, I feel bad and guilty; when I don't, I feel angry and cheated. I'm a wreck! I can't understand—smokers can conceive, selfish

*people can conceive, thieves can conceive. Why is an
honest, compassionate, generous, compulsive runner like
me being punished?*

A common response to feelings of guilt is the use of bargaining.
The person tries to atone for imaginary sins in order to receive
forgiveness in the form of a baby. This may be one of the reasons
infertility patients are willing to go to any length in order to conceive, including suffering through painful tests, surgery, and elaborate treatments. They may feel they are "purging" themselves.

To handle guilt, it is important first to recognize that feelings of
self-blame are a common, normal response to infertility. Even if full-
fledged guilt is not experienced, regrets often are ("I know I wasn't
ready to have kids ten years ago, but sometimes I wish I'd done it
anyhow"). Once you realize how common self-blame is, you may feel
less threatened by the feeling. A second step in handling guilt is
realizing that infertility has nothing to do with your worthiness as a
person. Intellectually, you may know this to be true, but do you
actually believe it? Sharing your guilty feelings with a close and
trusted friend and allowing that person to point out the unreality of
your self-blame can be helpful in dispelling these feelings.

Many people, though, are plagued by the belief that they are
being punished. Often, this conclusion again is the result of rigid
religious training that stressed the outcomes of "right" and "wrong"
behavior. If this is true of you, it may be necessary to reevaluate your
religious beliefs with a minister or counselor. Handling guilt means
coming to terms with what you really feel regarding painful issues in
the past and then learning to accept who you really are—a human
being with strengths and weaknesses.

ISOLATION

Isolation is another frequent response during this stage of the infertility process when testing and treatment are ruling your life. Although there is more openness these days, even regarding sex,
infertility still remains a secret issue—it can be embarrassing and
shameful to those experiencing it. So one tends to withdraw, to hide.

Contact with the world where signs of fertility are common
may also be painful. Infertile individuals often isolate themselves
from others, spending much time in solitary activity and avoiding
anything that involves children. Differences in life-styles, from that of

couples with children, can create more distance. Those with children are less free, and their activities change into family events. Thus there is less in common between those with and those without offspring.

> *I have almost totally cut off contact with a girlfriend I've been close to since childhood. She has one child and is pregnant again. We were once able to share so much. Our life experiences paralleled each other. Now she has child-related experiences and spends time with other young mothers. Many other friends have also begun to start families. We no longer socialize with them, as they are not as free to do the things we do.*

Of course, this kind of experience is natural for any childless couple, infertile or not, but the distance is more acutely felt by those who would like, but are unable, to have children.

As we will see in the chapter on social issues, it is not unusual for infertile people to alter their life-styles dramatically—anything to avoid contact with the world of fertility. This particular change, though, will not solve your problems. The loss of relationships with friends and family can be enormous. Most infertile people eventually find that they are better helped by establishing good communication with others and finding support from those who are experiencing similar difficulties with infertility. This is not the easy answer but, in the long run, it provides the best results.

DEPRESSION

Finally, the assault stage of infertility is likely to bring periods of depression, still another normal response to the pain of being infertile. Many are surprised by the strength of the emotional impact of their condition and by how depressed or anxious they have become.

> *Depression has been the most difficult emotion for me to handle, especially at night when I am trying to fall asleep. I have stopped working because, contrary to popular belief, working does not "take my mind off of it." I think about my infertility all the time. I am obsessed with it, am gaining weight, and not leading a very productive life. (Pardon the pun.)*

*There are so many days when it's difficult to keep back
the tears. Some days it feels like a lifelong obsession
that will not go away. Generally, on the surface it has
not affected my daily activities, but it has greatly
increased feelings of stress and has lessened my ability
to deal rationally with life's minor inconveniences.*

*For a long time, I have had to push myself to keep
functioning. I would never commit suicide, but often I
have wished that I would get hit by a truck so I
wouldn't have to endure it anymore.*

*When my period comes, I get into bed and just stay
there. I lose my ambition and ponder the futility of life.
I think about death a lot for the first time. I'm not even
enthusiastic about buying our first home. The real estate
brokers keep pushing cute little houses just right for
two adults. I can't stand it.*

Thoughts about death are common during the infertility struggle as people are brought face to face with their own mortality. You
may begin to feel very old, dwelling on the significance of yourself
in the passage of generations and worrying that you will not be able
to create an extension of yourself that will live on. One man described it this way:

*What infertility seemed to do for me was to force a
kind of confrontation with lifelessness or death. The
fact that there would be no children meant that I was
the last line of offense against death. Nobody to carry
on who was living. The solution: disconnect. So I
numbed out. I invested back into work, which in the
culture has been* man's *traditional way to combat
mortality. If your* work *lives on, you haven't been
wasting your time; there's a purpose to your life. . . . On
the other hand, [women's] infertility leaves them
defenseless, embodying the lifelessness even more and
without a culturally accepted avenue like "work" to
turn to.[2]*

Fears of death will often surface, in both men and women, during this period of depression.

Mild depression is a feeling of sadness or despair indicated by a loss of spontaneity, a feeling of malaise, tearfulness, loss of interest in normal activities, constant fatigue, and pessimistic thoughts. Everything takes extra effort to be accomplished and nothing seems as pleasurable as in the past. The mildly depressed person may be able to "put on a show" at work or in social situations, but close friends will notice differences in behavior. Some describe themselves as robots just going through the motions, but without life or feeling. Others become disorganized and apathetic about getting anything done; housework may go by the wayside and personal care may diminish. Often the person feels "defective"—ugly, sexually inadequate, incompetent, undesirable. This loss of self-esteem can extend to other areas of life, too, so that you feel a sense of failure in the workplace, for example.

If more severe depression develops, physical illnesses may occur and a feeling of gloom or hopelessness predominates. Some people become rundown and lethargic with slower bodily functions (thought processes, speech, motor functioning); others display severe anxiety or agitation. Common symptoms include persistent insomnia or early morning awakening, weight loss, and somatic complaints like gastrointestinal problems or general aches and pains. Serious depression can hide other strong emotions that the person is unable to handle. It is not unusual, for example, for the depressed person to be plagued by guilt or an intense sense of unworthiness.

Depression may be long lasting, often occurring throughout much of the treatment process. People cope with it in a variety of ways, some positive, some negative. Not uncommonly, people respond to depression by spending excessive amounts of money or by self-medicating with increased use of alcohol. These are only momentary solutions, however, and will simply increase the depression. It is far better to confront the painful feelings of sadness or anger inside you and find appropriate ways to express them—talking with others (your spouse, a close friend or relative), keeping a journal, or joining a support group. Bottling up your feelings will only make matters worse. If you recognize signs of serious depression in yourself and feel unable to control them, get professional help. It may be frightening to take this step, but the anxiety will eventually disappear and you will be glad you made the effort.

Because the condition of infertility is so inexact with no clear-cut end, depression can continue indefinitely, so that the grieving process never really starts. As will be discussed in the chapter "The Crossroads of Infertility," it is easy to get stuck in the mire of long-term depression and fail to move on toward resolution. Don't let this happen to you.

The Grieving Process

When conception has not occurred and a couple is considering ending treatment, a grieving process usually begins. Hope has disappeared and you mourn the child you will not have. During this phase and the next, a serious look at the meaning of parenthood takes place. An exploration of the parenting role will be more thoroughly addressed in the "Crossroads" chapter.

The grief reaction, or mourning process, is characterized by a number of behaviors:

1. Physical responses—sobbing, shortness of breath, tightness in the throat

2. Attempts to make sense of the loss; feelings of guilt

3. Emotional distance from others, characterized by withdrawal or anger

4. A sense of unreality

5. A change in normal behavior patterns; difficulty paying attention or remembering, lack of motivation, jumpiness

6. Constant preoccupation with thoughts of having a baby

Many of these behaviors may have occurred earlier in your response to infertility, but they will probably be repeated with intensity at this point. Grieving differs from prolonged depression in that it consists of acutely painful episodes of sobbing and despair. It is a well-documented, predictable chain of events that is essential to the resolution process. And, believe it or not, it does end. The problem is, however, that grief may be triggered monthly until it is substantially worked through.

It is important to recognize that infertility does not simply mean the loss of a baby. It is a complicated series of losses that strike deeply at the heart of the individual: the loss of a biological heir, loss of the physical experience of pregnancy and birth, loss of the breast-feeding experience, loss of a life goal, loss of a love child you and your spouse have conceived together, loss of self-esteem, loss of a sexual image of yourself, and loss of control.

The depth and extent of the losses will differ from one person to the next, depending on many factors. The most important are:

1. The quality of the marital relationship: Do you find your marriage to be a source of strength and support? Does the relationship with your spouse bring pleasure to you?

2. The degree of support from significant others: Do you have friends and relatives who are understanding and supportive? Are you able to confide in them?

3. The effectiveness of your personal coping skills: Have you developed a repertoire of coping mechanisms that can be counted on to help you through difficult times? Do you keep working on new skills?

4. The sensitivity of physicians: Do you feel comfortable with your physician? Do you find him or her to be sensitive to your emotional needs?

5. Your level of self-esteem to begin with: Did you have a positive self-image and a sense of confidence prior to learning of your infertility?

6. The extent of areas of strength in your life: Do you feel competent at work? Do you have interests that are pleasurable and satisfying?

If you have always felt negative about yourself and have few other strengths and supports in your life, this loss will be more difficult to accept.

If, when asking yourself these questions, you recognize that most of these factors are against you, it is time for some changes. Infertility will be devastating to most who experience it, but you do not need to endure it with three strikes against you. Begin to assess where you need help and support—from your spouse, from family and friends, through the way you are handling the situation? The remaining chapters will help you clarify these issues and will offer you, as an individual and as a couple, multiple strategies for change.

Acceptance/Resolution

Two of the most common statements you hear from those entering this stage are "It's time to move on" and "Enough is enough." This is the point when you make the personal decisions concerning the resolution of your crisis and your life plan. Behavioral changes are usually apparent, including improved self-esteem, more organized behavior, a resumption of social contacts, and a happier mood. It is a significant milestone. Reaching acceptance does not mean that you come to feel that your infertility is just or fair, only that you have faced its reality and have decided to go on living. Nor does it mean that painful feelings about infertility will be gone forever—they will surface again every once in a while. But they no longer run your life. The critical elements in acceptance and resolution are discussed in full detail in the last two chapters of the book.

Men vs. Women—Their Reactions to Infertility

Men's and women's feelings regarding infertility may not be too different, but their manner of expression and coping mechanisms can differ significantly. In past studies, most of the attention has focused on the female emotional reaction, while the male response has been largely ignored. The reasons are twofold. First, reproduction historically has been considered a female issue and any difficulties with conception were believed to be female in origin. Not being able to bear children was seen as a blow only to the woman because she would be unfulfilled. Second, most men have been taught to hide their tears; any display of sadness is a sign of weakness. Men are supposed to be strong and in control. It is not that they suffer less from infertility, only that they are less able to express emotion. Unfortunately, this means that men are often perceived as unaffected by the circumstance of infertility. They will exhibit a cool detachment that may belie their intense feelings, while women will openly cry in distress.

The following comments came from women telling how they and their spouses responded to infertility:

My husband is fairly stoic; I cry a lot.

I cry, talk about it, and let all the anxiety out. My

*husband keeps it inside and tries to get me to keep
things inside, too.*

*I am a worrier, so I tend to pick the situation to pieces
and examine every aspect. My husband does not readily
deal with problems. If something hurts him, he pushes
it to the back of his mind. As a result, I want to talk
about it much more than he does.*

*I know my husband feels sad, but he responds with
silence. I, on the other hand, am constantly ventilating.*

*I've become obsessed and vocal. My husband has
become even more quiet.*

This pattern often places the husband in a supportive role; he
exhibits quiet strength and attempts to restore equilibrium. Whatever he may be feeling is given little opportunity to be vented. Many
men will even say that they are concerned only because of their
wife's distress. When questioned at RESOLVE meetings or upon entering counseling, a man often states that he has come only because of
his wife's pushing him or because he "will do anything" to help her
feel better. Defenses, particularly denial, tend to be exceptionally
strong.

Even when the man has the primary medical problem, his denial
of the difficulty can be powerful. Experience may indicate there is
little possibility of conception because of low sperm count or poor
motility, but unless a diagnosis of azoospermia (no sperm) is made,
there is no clear-cut certainty about his infertility. Since there is
always the outside chance that conception could occur, it may be
hard for the male patient to come to grips with the reality of his
problem.

A strong handicap for men is the lack of opportunities to discuss
their feelings with peers. Because public expression of their emotions is so hard for men, they feel alone and different; they are
unaware there are many others out there suffering as they are. The
men with an actual medical problem (especially when their wives
hve gotten clean bills of health) are the loneliest of all and suffer the
most stress, for they have few, if any, supports.

My husband becomes very depressed over his infertility,

> *but refuses to talk about it. Several years ago, he broke*
> *a window in a rage after finding out I had gotten my*
> *period. His arm was all cut up, and he didn't even*
> *remember what he had done the minute before. He gets*
> *very depressed whenever infertility is mentioned on*
> *television. He thinks he's the only one with this problem*
> *and is always asking God what he did to deserve this.*

In cases in which the medical difficulty is the woman's, the man may not realize for a long time that his life, not just his wife's, has been affected by the problem of infertility. At some point, though, men do begin to notice the effects on themselves—constant tension, irritability at work, pangs of envy when they watch fathers and their children, or out-of-proportion sadness when they hear unhappy news. Since crying is not often acceptable and infertility does not represent a "concrete" loss, grieving becomes very difficult. Men are likely to throw themselves into their work, struggling to push painful feelings away.

> *"[As] a man, I could block the problem quite*
> *efficiently, at least on the surface. I felt angry at my*
> *powerlessness and at the unhappiness it was causing*
> *my wife. But I could block, and work, and survive."*[3]

Although men are hindered from experiencing the mourning process, it is as necessary for them as for women. Male discomfort with emotions and the failure to mourn present a major problem in marital decision making about infertility issues. It is one reason women often feel prepared for inquiring into alternatives at an earlier point than do their husbands, a situation that can lead to conflict.

> *My husband has never been one to talk about problems*
> *and that had been okay so far, but this problem needed*
> *discussing. He just couldn't see that there was anything*
> *to be so upset over (I am the infertile one). He thought*
> *everything would work out in the end, that I would*
> *become pregnant. It took him longer to come to the*
> *decision to adopt and that frustrated me.*

Understanding Each Other's Reactions

Timing will rarely be synchronized, but if husbands are given greater opportunity to explore and share their feelings along the way, it is likely there will be less discrepancy in the amount of time each spouse takes to approach new interventions on the road to resolution. As a woman, you should ask yourself how you felt in the past when you had a problem and your husband came home with a problem, too: did you feel cheated or disappointed not to have his full attention and support? Did you perhaps unconsciously expect him always to be the strong one? It is easy for partners to slip into this pattern of the wife as "ventilator" and the husband as "Rock of Gibraltar." Wives can assist their husbands by avoiding becoming so focused on themselves that they cannot see beyond their own emotional turmoil. They can also help by asking questions, encouraging discussion, not expecting their husbands always to be a pillar of strength. Support groups for individuals (men or women) and couples can be helpful here, too.

Since men and women do express themselves in different ways, it is crucial to be both sensitive to and accepting of these differences. Although tears and verbal expressions of grief are probably most effective in working through painful feelings of loss, many find other ways of accomplishing this task. Some people (especially men), for example, throw themselves into vigorous physical activity as a catharsis for strong emotion. Because of their husband's silence, many women are misled to believe they are not experiencing sadness or dealing with their grief; but words are not always necessary.

Both partners need to be patient in resolving their dissimilar ways of reacting. The tendency is for frustration to mount, with each spouse standing firm (Wife: "We need to talk"; Husband: "There's nothing to talk about"). The distance between them becomes greater. But barriers like this can be worked through with effort from both sides. The suggestions in the chapter "Infertility and the Couple" may help you.

Reactions Spouses Share

With regard to actual feelings, there is probably less discrepancy between men and women. Both may feel defective or unworthy, with these feelings spilling over into other areas of life.

*My self-esteem has very much lowered, although I don't
believe it shows outwardly. It's an internal feeling of
inadequacy. I feel like I'm imperfect, unable to do what
other men seem to accomplish effortlessly.*

*I never dreamed I would ever have difficulty in
achieving what I thought was the reason I was put on
earth for. My self-esteem right now is very low and I
feel useless both as a woman and as a wife. I feel like
a factory irregular.*

*I always dreamed of being a mother and have not yet
found my purpose in life. My life is empty. I weigh
more today than ever. I am a homebody, not visiting
certain friends or family. My character has changed on
the job. I am very aware of what I say before I speak.
Everything seems difficult for me. Nothing is that
important anymore.*

Men, initially, may feel that their knowledge of sex or their
ability to "perform" is inadequate. The lessening of sexual interest
during infertility can exacerbate the man's feeling that he lacks viril-
ity or masculinity. On occasion, a man may resort to casual affairs
with women who know nothing of his infertility problem in order to
prove to himself that he is still desirable.

Women, on the other hand, often report feelings of emptiness,
or a sense of being incomplete. They may feel unattractive or dis-
figured, even though the condition is not noticeable to others.

*Infertility has greatly affected my self-esteem and
self-image. My body no longer pleases me and the scars
from extensive surgery are a daily reminder of my
body's betrayal. I view my body as a traitor in that it
has not been able to nurture a pregnancy, nor will it
allow me to become pregnant again.*

*I have needed to reevaluate myself as a "whole woman."
Infertility did not affect my ability to enjoy
lovemaking, but I hated myself—my body for failing
me. It angered me that I could not control the "house I*

live in"—my body. It has made me humble as a human
being and made me realize the frailty of human lives.

Self-esteem? I have none because of my infertility. I feel
that I'm not quite a total woman. I see myself as
unfeminine and never feel pretty, although physically
I'm an okay-looking woman.

Many women, like men, feel that they must be sexually undesirable
and that their sexual functioning is inadequate or abnormal. Some
say that they no longer feel like part of the female sex, that they are
an "it" without the capacity to reproduce.

I have always been in conflict about my femaleness
and, being infertile, confirmed my worst suspicions that
I was biologically inadequate, hairier than others, and,
in general, more masculine than I should be. In
addition, my husband's development of a problem with
impotence fed into my worries that I was an
unattractive woman and undesirable.

The negative side effects of many infertility drugs (weight gain, acne,
nausea) can exacerbate your dissatisfaction with your body.

To compound the problem, some women consider pregnancy
and birth to be the highest evidence of maturity—thus, failure to
reproduce is perceived as a lack of psychosexual development and a
defect of their womanhood. In contrast, reproduction, for many
men, is only secondary to career development and being a good
provider. It may be easier, then, for a man to find other avenues for
obtaining self-esteem.

For both men and women, however, negative feelings about
oneself, even those that have been worked through in the past, can
often resurface as a result of infertility.

I have always struggled with low self-esteem and now
feel that I have failed in a very important way by not
having a baby. Starting to go through the adoption
process doesn't help this a whole lot either because you
have to prove to them that you would be a good parent
and worthy of a child. I work in a clinic where I see, at

*times, neglected and abused children who the courts try
to keep with their natural families and I wonder why
it's okay for them to have children and not for me and
my husband. Intellectually, I understand the process, but
emotionally it means something else. I was abused as a
child and was always afraid of the prophecy of an
abused child growing up to be an abusive parent. I
worked my whole life to get rid of the effects of my
childhood, but infertility seems to make all the old
feelings come right back.*

When this occurs, it does not mean that all your previous work was
in vain—only that your psychological gains have been challenged
and need to be strengthened.

Finally, for both men and women, even a basic outlook on life
can drastically change as a result of the experience of infertility.

*I was always a basically optimistic person who believed
that things would work out okay in the end. I also
believed that there was a reason for all of life's bad
experiences. Now I'm more of a pessimist and have
become more negative about many things. Sometimes I
even question now whether I would be a good parent,
when before I was sure I would be.*

Although this is a painful time to weather, most do find that their
previous optimism and satisfaction with life eventually return, once
resolution has been reached.

Is There a Psychological Basis to Infertility?

Only twenty years ago, it was believed that as much as 40 percent of
all infertility problems had a psychological origin.[4] At that time, a
psychogenic diagnosis was frequently made when no physical cause
could be determined. Since the field was relatively unsophisticated,
large numbers of infertile people were left with the understanding
that their emotional conflicts were the culprit. This is certainly a far
cry from today's 10 percent of cases with unexplained medical
causes, but unfortunately the belief persists that emotional factors

lead to infertility. Noting the frequency of the advice to "relax!" can give you some idea of how prevalent this idea still is.

As we have noted, the blame for psychogenic infertility historically has been placed upon the woman. During earlier years, studies compared fertile and infertile individuals, predominantly women, and came up with a cluster of personality factors that were regarded as typical of the infertile person. One study suggested that infertile couples exhibited more ambivalence about children than those with proven fertility, and another investigation noted that "psychogenic infertility could be considered a defense against dangers inherent in the reproductive function." Other studies purported to show that infertile women were struggling with issues regarding their femininity and that both infertile men and women might have "various psychosexual maladjustments."[5] All this seems rather strange when you consider the very anxious, even emotionally unstable, people who have had no difficulty whatever conceiving.

Other research, however, contrary to these studies, has found no correlation between psychological problems and infertility. The reason for the discrepancy in results is most likely due to the fact that the stress of infertility can *lead* to emotional problems; if this is not taken into account, erroneous causal factors for infertility might be implied. Researchers have been unable to show that emotional difficulties apparent in infertile couples are the cause of, rather than the result of, infertility.[6]

As further evidence, studies on postadoptive conception have been reviewed by Seibel and Taylor, in their article "Emotional Aspects of Infertility," and they state that "statistical evidence is overwhelmingly against the relationship of adoption and subsequent conception."[7] This, too, indicates the tenuous, and probably nonexistent, causal relationship between emotions and infertility.

The effect of erroneous psychogenic diagnoses made in the past has been problematic in several respects. First, it created additional guilt and depression in infertile individuals who were already facing significant stress. Second, it misled the public and encouraged negative perceptions and comments. Third, it made people hesitant to seek counseling regarding the normal stresses of infertility for fear that they would be blamed for their difficulties. When others respond with "Don't worry so much" or "Are you sure you *really* want to have children?" it is very hard not to dwell on these thoughts. As John Stangel states in *Fertility and Conception*, being told not to worry is like being told not to think about your breathing—you can then do nothing else.

Although no case has been made for psychogenic infertility, it is important to realize that infertility can cause stress and stress can certainly have an effect on physiological processes. It does not appear to inhibit conception on an ongoing basis, but it can interfere temporarily. For example, tension might lead to a man developing temporary impotence or a woman experiencing difficulty with penetration during intercourse. Stress can also negatively affect the number and motility of sperm in the male or inhibit ovulation in the female, though these were not initially identified as problems contributing to a couple's infertility. Stangel notes that stress might, in addition, cause some discoordination of the fallopian tubes in "certain very limited circumstances."[8] He concludes, however, by emphasizing the decreasing use of the psychogenic diagnosis and the low probability that stress has much of an impact on conception.

Some people, unfortunately, tear themselves apart thinking that their emotional state is causing their infertility. This is counterproductive. If you do have genuine concerns about becoming a parent or about your sexuality, then consider getting help in resolving them. But recognize that these worries have not been proven to cause infertility. Emotional issues, whether contributing to or resulting from infertility, need to be dealt with as an adjunct to medical treatment. Even if anxiety is not a primary cause, it might prevent the body from functioning most effectively.

Most stressful is the predicament of unexplained infertility. In this situation, a couple has undergone a thorough evaluation and no medical cause has been determined—they are part of the 10 percent of cases noted earlier. Occasionally, these people are described as "normal" infertile couples, which is misleading because they are clearly not normal. They are unable to conceive, and they are struggling as much as any other infertile couple, but their problem is as yet unexplained.

> *The uncertainty of it all, the lack of a clear diagnosis, is excruciating. I never know whether I'm being realistic or pessimistic. Getting my hopes up and then grieving—every month. That's a killer! Lately I've just been feeling helpless and exhausted. I don't understand it at all, and there are no answers.*

In the past, these couples might have been told they were having psychological problems that were interfering with reproduction. Now it is believed that science is not yet sophisticated enough to identify what the physiological difficulty is—there are limits to medical knowledge, despite its progress. As a result, these situations tend to be major frustrations for both couples and physicians alike. Being told of a specific problem that is causing infertility is a blow, but at least it is a concrete reality that can be faced and worked through. Not knowing the cause means that the couple must continue to struggle with uncertainty. It is a maddening situation. If pregnancy does not eventually occur, it can be exceptionally difficult to stop the struggle and consider other options for resolution.

Infertility takes a tremendous toll on the lives of infertile people with overwhelming physical, financial, and emotional pressures. Becoming a parent is a major life accomplishment denied to many couples. It can be a crisis of enormous magnitude that propels entire lives into disequilibrium. Understand that the feelings described in this chapter are normal responses to this crisis and that they are not indicative of mental illness, even though you may sometimes feel like you're going off the deep end. Don't be any harder on yourself than the situation already is.

Infertile in a
Fertile Society

One of the most difficult aspects of being infertile is learning to face and relate to a fertile world. There is no escaping it. Whether you are shopping at the grocery store, handling the responsibilities of your job, or just watching television (with the inevitable Pampers commercials), you will be confronted with painful reminders of your infertility. Suddenly you avoid or are uncomfortable with fertile friends, relatives, or colleagues with whom you had good relationships in the past. A Saturday evening get-together that was so enjoyable before infertility entered your life becomes a chore because of the constant fear that the topic of children might arise. Holidays with your family are no longer times of celebration but, instead, times that are dreaded long before they arrive. Pregnant women and babies suddenly seem to be jumping out of the woodwork everywhere you turn. Even if you make a valiant attempt to hibernate, it will be impossible totally to escape the impact of a fertile society.

Relating to the Fertile World

It is not easy for the infertile person to deal with others in the fertile world, but it is also not easy for those others to know how to deal with infertility. Everyone has his or her own particular personality and set of needs, and it can be difficult to know what is best for each person. Many infertile couples, for example, complain that their friends or family are too nosy, too intrusive ("I wish they'd leave us alone. Don't they know that if there's any news, we'll send up fireworks!"). Others complain with equal intensity that their loved ones never ask any questions and seem uncaring or disinterested ("They don't seem to give a damn about us. How can they not recognize the agony we're going through?"). To complicate matters, the infertile person's needs often change; sometimes one needs to discuss the problem obsessively and, other times, one wants to avoid the issue altogether. Only you, as an individual, can identify the style that you are most comfortable with and that best suits your needs at a given time. Although it is difficult, it is your responsibility to clarify for others what is helpful and comforting and what is not.

The following discussion suggests ways for handling infertility that you can adjust to fit your personality and needs. It is always *your* choice with whom you communicate and how much you decide to share. But, remember, friends and family are important and can be a valuable asset while you are struggling through infertility.

Facing Yourself

Before you begin work on relating to others, you must first examine the attitude you have toward yourself and your infertility. Many see it as an embarrassment or a shame that must be hidden. This poses a problem because as long as you view infertility as a negative reflection on yourself (your character or your sexuality) you are asking for a negative response from others. You are your own worst enemy. How can you ask others to accept and understand your condition for what it is—a medical problem—if you yourself are ashamed?

> *I hated myself at first. I felt useless as a woman and just wanted to hide. I can remember, only too well, wanting a hysterectomy. If the parts aren't working, why have them?*

> *Because I can't tell people about my infertility, I definitely must have a problem with self-esteem though I tell myself I don't. I know infertility shouldn't be shameful, but I dread the day when our small town of three hundred people knows the truth.*

It is important to ask yourself: Why are you feeling so embarrassed or ashamed? How do you think others' perceptions of you would change if they knew of your problem?

The public holds many misconceptions about infertility and cannot be expected to attain a more realistic understanding if the problem is shrouded in embarrassment and secrecy. If you can talk openly about the issue, even on an intellectual level, you have made an important move forward. For example, tell those close to you about your diagnosis and the available treatments—give them the medical knowledge you are beginning to learn. It is a first step toward helping others accept your situation and will break down the isolation that so frequently accompanies the infertility experience.

Exploring Your Feelings in Social Situations

"Do you have any children?" A simple but often painful question, it rapidly brings into focus all the hurt you feel and contrasts it sharply with the joys perceived in the fertile world. The question is likely to produce an explosion of feelings inside you, and you won't know how to respond. It is important to become aware of how you are feeling in various social environments, especially those that confront your infertility head-on (at a baby shower or when a friend tells you that she is pregnant). It may be very difficult to accept the feelings that are flourishing within you—the hatred, rage, envy—especially if you have always thought of yourself as a nice person and a good friend.

> *I would walk down the street and every time that I saw a pregnant woman I had the sudden fantasy of punching her in the belly. Both as a health care professional and as a moral person, I found these feelings of rage and aggression hard to tolerate within myself.*

The fact is you are entitled to your feelings. Infertility hurts and there is no point in trying to deny the pain. It is the *not* allowing yourself to feel that can cause trouble because it prevents you from working through the crisis to a healthy resolution.

When a friend tells you that she is pregnant, accept the fact that, at best, your feelings toward her will be ambivalent. More than likely, you will be consumed by intense jealousy.

> *A friend and I had experienced years of infertility together and were major supports for one another. Then*

*the day arrived when she told me that she was
pregnant—I'll never forget it. I wanted to be happy for
her and tried to feel encouraged by her success, but I
didn't. Jealousy raged within me and the tears just kept
streaming down my cheeks. The first day that she wore
a maternity dress I thought I would die on the spot. She
had everything I wanted and I couldn't bear to look at
her. Even worse, I felt that I had lost my strongest
support.*

Understand too that when others talk of their ease in becoming
pregnant or their unhappiness in having conceived unexpectedly
that you will probably feel bitter and cheated. There's nothing
wrong in feeling that way.

Finally, recognize that you may have an extreme sensitivity to
pregnancy-related issues that is hard to control in public and that is
likely to affect your ability to relate to others. You may also be
constantly on guard, anticipating uncomfortable situations and carrying a chip on your shoulder.

*Pregnancy was so much on my mind that I became
acutely perceptive in identifying the possible signs in
myself and others. Even before pregnancies were
announced and no one else had an inkling of the
situation, I often was aware of others being pregnant.
Little signs, invisible to most, stood out like beacons to
me. For example, when my sister was only two weeks
pregnant and hadn't even had a pregnancy test yet
(although she suspected she was with child), I "knew"
about it. I noticed during that visit that she chose to
drink soda, not wine, and that one morning she went
back to bed "not feeling well." Other minor cues leapt
out at me and I grew increasingly depressed without
one word about pregnancy ever being mentioned. For
the rest of the visit, I acted like a zombie and no one
even knew why.*

"No One Understands"

Many of you may handle the intense feelings surrounding your infertility by shutting them off and withdrawing from family and friends.

Some couples will dramatically change their life-style—quit jobs, move, terminate friendships—to avoid anything that reminds them of children. Isolating yourself from others who seem to be happy with their lives is common, and when you are infertile, anyone with children may be perceived as being happy. Everyone knows that's not true, but who is being rational?

Most of you probably want others to understand the depth of your despair, but if you close them out, you give them little opportunity. This leads to the frequent complaint, "No one understands." Unless you share some of the pressures you are under, others, who cannot read your mind, will not know what you are experiencing. Remember, no one, especially fertile friends, can really share the impact of your crisis because it affects each individual in a different way. If you stop expecting others to understand completely what you are feeling and just seek their acceptance and support, you will make it much easier for yourself.

It is not unusual, especially for a woman, to become obsessed with infertility and the desire to become pregnant. It is easy to develop a "fishbowl" existence, becoming blind to all other problems in life, and focusing only on your own little world of pain. But others are experiencing their own life crises—health problems, loss of loved ones, economic stresses, marital discord. It is unfair to expect them to feel your intense pain, just as you are feeling it, when they may be struggling with their own problems. Moreover, if you are too obsessed with infertility, others may be tired of hearing about it.

On occasion, people will jump to inaccurate conclusions about your childlessness, perhaps insinuating that you must be a career person with no interest in children or that your marriage is too unstable for starting a family. These comments may make you furious, and certainly they would have been better left unsaid, but if you want other people to understand the situation accurately, only you can set them straight. You might say, for example, "What you've just said isn't at all true. We love children and want very much to start a family. Unfortunately, though, we've been having some medical problems." Whether you then decide to pursue the subject further would depend on how interested the person is and how comfortable you feel.

A frequent obstacle in accurate communication about infertility is the person putting on a brave front—the "stiff upper lip" syndrome. Many of you will do this throughout your infertility, and, at times, it is a necessity. But remember that acting this way *all* the time may give others a distorted perception of how you are feeling. If you volunteer to give a baby shower for a friend or question your sister about the details of her pregnancy, how is anyone going to know how upsetting these events are for you? They cannot understand your hurt and be sensitive to your predicament when all signs indicate that you are managing quite well.

Sharing Feelings

Five and a half years ago, one of my friends had her first child. She was frightened and ambivalent about the pregnancy and the experience was difficult for both of us. The day before she delivered, we had lunch and spoke of how we wished we could be having babies together. We shared as best we could. One year later, when we very suddenly adopted our daughter, my friend was there with the baby clothes and the instructions. The following year we both became pregnant, celebrated together, and miscarried within a week of each other. Thirteen months after our miscarriages, we each delivered our second child. My friend and I have shared childbearing and child rearing in all its forms and it has definitely enriched our relationship. We love to reflect back on each of the steps along the way and to marvel at the wonderful and mysterious ways in which families are born.

As difficult as it may sound, it is important to try to tell those closest to you some of the feelings you have. The woman who contributed the experience related above benefited from a very special relationship because she was able to share her feelings, rather than closing off. If, at first, it seems impossible to talk freely, it may help to offer family or close friends an article on infertility or a RESOLVE newsletter to open up the discussion. If you feel totally unable to share with others in your life, it may be easier to join an organization like RESOLVE. There is a camaraderie, an instant understanding, within an infertility support organization that can make communication more comfortable and give you practice for opening up to others in your life. Many people find that after they have taken that first difficult step in sharing feelings or experiences they feel less alone and victimized.

I have become very open about my infertility over time. Keeping it a secret only magnified the problem, so admitting it has been somewhat of a release. It has continued to hurt when sharing it with close friends who have just announced a pregnancy, but keeping close-mouthed was worse.

Once my husband and I began telling others of our difficulty, it felt like a great burden had been lifted. Friends and family suddenly began to contact us with news about infertility that they had seen on television or read in the paper. Had we heard about the latest new development? Some people might have considered this an intrusion, especially if the information had little to do with their specific problem, but we found it to be comforting. It allowed others to feel that they were offering some help and it let us know that they cared.

In sharing feelings with others, honesty is usually the best route to take. If friends have a baby and keep inviting you to their home, a situation you find intolerable, then let them know about your discomfort. Most people will understand that, although you care for them, it is too painful to be around their child right now. If you avoid the issue, your feelings are likely to surface as aloof, anxious behavior which may then be misinterpreted.

If you find yourself needing more space, especially from a pregnant friend, again, try to share those feelings. Let your friend know that you need some time to deal with your sadness and envy. Of course, some people will be angry or offended by your honesty, but in my experience most try to understand the situation. And if they don't understand completely, they will at least be more aware of your predicament. Again, others cannot know what hurts unless you tell them.

Remember that the manner in which you communicate your feelings is crucial. If you have been storing up anger and then suddenly blast someone for what you perceive to be insensitivity, you will not get a very positive response. Share your thoughts in a direct but tactful manner without overtones of aggression.

I haven't been very open about my infertility. I tried to be but failed miserably at it and all of my relationships have been affected. I've been impatient, intolerant of dumb remarks, very emotional, easily hurt, and distant. People have been afraid to approach me because they didn't know what to say or what reaction they'd get.

Unfortunately, one of the hazards in opening up about your infertility is that others may respond with pity, rather than understanding. It can be very uncomfortable to have others feel sorry for you. If that happens, try to take control of the situation by explaining what helps and what does not.

Being Prepared

Social situations in which you are caught offguard are inevitable, so it is helpful to think ahead and prepare for encounters that are likely to happen. For example, consider the stock questions people often ask when first meeting someone:

Do you have any children?

Are you planning to have a family?

Where do your children go to school?

Even more painful is someone's attempt to pursue a conversation about children with a remark like "You really should think about starting a family. Kids are wonderful!" It helps to be prepared with some ideas for automatic responses because the anxiety these questions engender can make you instantly tongue-tied. If you need to, practice at home until you find a response that is comfortable. For example, if someone asks if you have children, you might simply say, "We're working on it!" or "No, but we're seriously thinking about it." If you want to share a little more, your response could be "We'd love to start a family but have had some difficulty."

If someone pushes the discussion of children to an uncomfortable point, learn the technique of "turning the tables." That means to take the offensive with questions or comments about *them*: "It really seems to bother you that we don't have children" or "It must have been hard for you to have given up your career to have kids." Let them get fidgety and defensive, instead of you.

You should also be aware ahead of time as to what events are going to be difficult for you to attend and make your plans accordingly.

> *My most difficult experience was an evening spent with two other couples who had children. The children, their mothers, and I were sitting in the living room. One of my friends was rocking her newborn to sleep, while the other was playing with her toddlers. I sat in a corner of the room watching all of this interaction. It was almost dreamlike. I suddenly realized how out-of-place I was . . . a sore thumb. I felt such hurt, loneliness, and a terrible sense of emptiness. As usual, I held my tears and my friends never suspected my pain that night. But it is an evening I'll never forget.*

Learning to decline invitations for stressful occasions like baby showers or birthday parties may be necessary. Or if a particular situation cannot be avoided, shortening your visit can be an alternative. Remember that if you are feeling terrible and you spend the occasion sitting alone in a corner, your behavior is likely to make everyone feel uncomfortable; you would have been better off not attending at all. These decisions, however, must be made on an individual basis since everyone's coping skills vary. If possible, try to be honest in giving explanations so that short stays or declined invitations are not misconstrued.

Handling Advice and Unwelcome Comments

> *"Don't worry—my cousin, Harriet, took ten months to conceive her third child."*

> *"You just need to relax. I bet a romantic vacation in the Caribbean would do the trick!"*

"Maybe you should adopt—then you're sure to get pregnant."

"I think you're just trying too hard. Don't think about it so much."

"You know, it's really not so bad. Just look at all the freedom you have while we're stuck home with the kids."

You have all heard and probably cringed at these unsolicited "words of wisdom." Unfortunately, as these comments suggest, the public is often misinformed about infertility. In other cases, comments are made by people who are so uncomfortable with the subject or with your pain that they offer advice that denies the existence of a problem. In either situation, it is difficult to be on the receiving end of these remarks and to know how to respond. In all likelihood, you have felt exasperated, furious, sad, or helpless—but said nothing. The problem with that reaction is it leads to isolation. What began as a medical problem with infertility has become compounded by silence and withdrawal—that is, if you allow it to happen.

Try to remember that when people make insensitive remarks or ask hurtful questions, it is not usually with malicious intent. More often it is just ignorance. Unsolicited advice may also arise out of anxiety. When friends are nervous and unsure of how to be helpful, they are likely to want to share whatever knowledge they have, no matter how misinformed. No one likes the feeling of helplessness. When inaccurate advice is offered, let people know that they are misinformed and provide them with correct information. Or you might say, "I know you're trying to help, but your comments make me more uncomfortable."

On occasion, you may encounter people who seem utterly unaware of how destructive their comments are:

"I guess that you just weren't meant to be a parent. It's God's will and He knows best."

"You probably aren't pregnant because of your conflict about having a family. There must be part of you that doesn't want children."

One hopes that outrageous comments like these will be few and far between, but you will hear some:

> *My sister-in-law has really added to our misery.*
> *Whenever we are with her, she casually brings up items*
> *like: "Gee, if you saw the beautiful maternity clothes*
> *out now, you'd go crazy" or "Everytime I see a new*
> *baby it makes me want to have another one" (as she*
> *nudges her husband's elbow for effect). This may sound*
> *horrible, but there have been several instances when I*
> *almost socked her, but being rather meek (and a good*
> *Christian) I laugh it off and hold my tears for the ride*
> *home.*

> *Last year I had a family party to celebrate the Fourth of*
> *July. In the middle of the party, my brother-in-law*
> *decided to tell all of the family how my husband and I*
> *reminded him of a "childless" pair of ducks (he called*
> *them Gertrude and Harry) that lived in his backyard. I*
> *had a very difficult time trying not to dissolve into*
> *tears. Thank goodness, no one else thought his cruel*
> *remarks were funny.*

> *My hardest experience with infertility came from an*
> *insensitive sister-in-law. My husband and I have had a*
> *wonderful Fresh Air child from New York City each*
> *summer for the past three years. At a party when she*
> *was sitting on my lap, my sister-in-law remarked in*
> *front of everyone that I was "pretending to be a*
> *mommy."*

Only you can decide how to manage such predicaments—do you confront these people or avoid them? Depending on who has made the remarks, you might try to make them understand. For example, you could say: "It really hurts when you make comments like that. We want to be parents more than anything in the world and have to struggle every day with tests and treatment. Can you imagine what it would be like if you'd never been able to have your children?" If this is unsuccessful, though, recognize that it is their problem, not yours.

There are occasions when you must protect yourself from painful situations, and this is one.

Relating to Your Family

Dealing with family members can be an intense experience when you are handling infertility. Every family has its own style for dealing with problems: some jump in head-first ready to find answers, whereas others never discuss personal issues. Both extremes can present problems but, judging from my clinical experience, it seems to be especially painful when family members are reluctant to talk and can't understand the devastating effect infertility has on the person's life.

> *My family and my husband's family favor denying the problem or, I should say, ignoring that this is something major in our lives. I know that both families are sad about it, but they don't want us to be sad so not talking about it seems best to them. I also think they're afraid my husband and I might separate because of our infertility problem, so they try to trivialize the situation.*

> *My parents are infertile—my brother and I were adopted after they tried for ten years to have a child. I thought my mother would really be understanding . . . WRONG! My father denies the whole issue and my mother just keeps saying, "Relax—you'll get pregnant." I now realize that they were never able to resolve their own infertility in their minds. They still have a lot of pain. I just want them to listen and be supportive. That hasn't happened yet.*

> *My parents and siblings act as if my infertility does not exist. They do not address it with me, and if there is any discussion, it is brought up by me. My Dad feels that for me to consider surrogate mothering or embryo transfer, instead of adopting, is the most selfish statement he has ever heard. He has no idea of how it*

hurts to not "feel" feminine because of not being able
to conceive. My Mom feels that adopting a child will
meet my every need and also ignores the issue of
pregnancy. All my brother and sister can say is "Well, at
least you can adopt." Everyone is quite uncomfortable
when I bring the subject up—I guess because they can't
change my situation. I just want them to acknowledge
my feelings as okay.

For some of you, this rift between you and your family may be
the most tragic consequence of infertility. Others who suffer are
individuals who have never had positive relationships with their
family and who look upon the birth of a child as their only means of
developing a new and satisfying sense of family. Even those who have
had close family ties may feel significant pain in "denying" their
parents a grandchild.

My father died in the midst of our infertility treatment.
That was one of the hardest times for me because I felt
that he had died without ever seeing a grandchild. I
was Daddy's girl and it was a very special relationship.
I wanted so much for him to experience the joy of a
grandchild and was tormented by my inability to share
this with him. Later, after we adopted, I took my
daughter to the cemetery to "meet" him and now I feel
he's had a chance to know her. I've gotten over it, but
it's taken some time.

Old conflicts with parents or siblings are often renewed after years
of compatibility, for example, when your siblings have children and a
resurgence of sibling rivalry develops. One of the most distressing
experiences in infertility can occur when a sister or sister-in-law
(almost always younger or certainly married for a shorter time)
becomes pregnant.

It tore me apart to watch my sister go through her
pregnancy and deliver a baby boy. I was so jealous that
it couldn't be me wearing that maternity dress and
having everyone lay their hand on my belly. She kept
getting all the attention, and inside I yearned to have

that attention too. I wanted to yell at everyone, "Don't be happy—it's not me!"

My younger sister had two children and was expecting another while I sat struggling month after month to conceive. Strangely, what hurt the most was that she kept naming her babies with the names I dreamed of using. We had never even discussed our favorites, but there it was—her "stealing" names from me. I silently screamed, "That's mine—you can't have it!" but never said a word.

You may even fear that your parents will not love you as much if you cannot bear grandchildren for them. These feelings may intensify if your parents seem to be focusing more attention on your sibling's family, eliciting envy and perhaps a sense of being deserted.

Sometimes comments from family members imply you are a failure for not producing children and providing genetic continuity. With or without such pressure, you may find that you are directing considerable anger at your parents in particular. You may assume they lack understanding, or you may even feel that they lied to you because they raised you with the belief that someday you would be a parent, just like them.

But your parents may be questioning how much they should intrude into your thoughts and emotions. What you may be reading as callousness, criticism, or disinterest may actually be their discomfort in not knowing what or how much to say. People in the throes of infertility tend to be defensive, or not uncommonly giving others the impression that they want no interference or communication whatsoever. It is always easier to blame your parents for lack of sensitivity than to recognize your own anxiety and distancing mechanisms. This is certainly not always true, but it is useful to explore your own behavior before jumping to conclusions, so that you do not project your own anxieties onto those you care for most.

When personal pain is so intense, it is often difficult for people to see beyond themselves, to recognize that others might also be suffering. Many parents are also grieving: over their children enduring pain and over their own loss of grandchildren.

My mother was the first person I told. She offered the

usual suggestions: "Relax"; "Don't think about it so much." She did not seem to understand how much I just needed to be comforted and to get validation of my feelings. But then I realized that she was hurting in response to my hurt. It was easier for her to quickly dismiss my feelings with "It will happen someday." It was her attempt at denial.

Although the feelings experienced by your parents may not be as intense as yours, they are not dissimilar; they too may feel shock, disappointment, frustration, anger, sadness. They may even feel a sense of guilt, wondering whether they contributed in any way to your infertility problem. One parent thought back to the drugs she took in order to prevent the miscarriage of a baby, now her infertile daughter, and wondered about their impact. Your parents, too, may have fantasized about the arrival of grandchildren, perhaps saving old toys and baby clothes to hand on to the next generation. When their friends become grandparents and begin proudly displaying "brag books," the feelings of envy, sadness, and disappointment may be strong. The same can be true when others raise questions about the likelihood of them having grandchildren. Parents may even share the same out-of-control feelings that you are experiencing. After all, parents are supposed to be able to dry those tears and make everything better. But infertility is not something they can put a Band-Aid on, nor is it just a financial problem they can help solve by offering money.

Remember that as you are working through your grieving process and approaching resolution, whether it be consideration of adoption, childfree living, or alternative means of biological parenting, your parents must also explore and deal with their own attitudes toward these options. The decisions are always yours in the end, but almost everyone will be facing some turmoil, too.

Some of you may recognize your parents' pain and for that reason be reluctant to open up.

My family and I have handled my infertility mostly with silence. I consider myself fortunate because there are no children as yet in our family, but I know my mother and mother-in-law (both widows) long for grandchildren. They seem to ache as I do and I find it

difficult to express my pain for fear of making it more
painful for them. I wish I could talk more openly with
them.

But talking rarely makes a situation more painful. It only opens doors
to sharing and closeness. Chances are that silent relatives, whom you
know to be caring and sensitive people, are yearning, like this young
woman, to communicate with you. They may even be hurt by your
decision not to share your feelings. It is likely, if you made an effort
to talk, that you would receive the support you so desperately need.

You should ask yourself whether you have really opened the
door for communication with your family or have erected invisible
walls. Just as the struggle with infertility can offer the opportunity
for growth for an individual or couple, it can also be the source of
growth for a family. Learning to communicate in a new and more
sensitive way over such an issue can provide tremendous rewards.

Coping with the Holidays

If you notice a slowly growing feeling of gloom within yourself as
the days shorten, the temperatures drop, and the leaves begin to fall,
it may simply be that you hate winter. But it is more likely that the
effects of the holiday season are already beginning to envelop you.
The holidays bombard everyone with pressures, but if you are infertile, the pressure may be overwhelming. On Halloween, you must
face all those giggling children arriving at your door with proud
parents watching in the background; then it is on to Thanksgiving
for a full dose of family togetherness and the need to give thanks
when inside you are feeling angry and deprived; and finally comes
the Hanukkah and Christmas season, the most pressure-packed of
them all.

Christmas and Hanukkah are especially difficult because the personal expectations that people have for these holidays are extremely
high. This season is a time of nostalgia, reviving memories of youth
and innocence that contrast sharply with present anger and disillusionment. For those with unhappy memories, the pressure may be
even greater because of the need to create a new life and a new
family that would erase childhood sadness. All people, whether experiencing infertility or not, have to face their own wishes for holiday perfection and the disappointment that invariably comes from

impossible fantasies. The child's-eye view of Christmas—in which the glittering tree seems so tall, the presents mountainous, and the excitement over Santa's arrival hard to contain—often stays with you as you fool yourself into thinking that personal difficulties will magically disappear. Many exert tremendous pressure on themselves to be joyous because it is a time when you are "supposed" to be rejoicing. If you recognize that you are not at all in a jovial mood, feelings of guilt and self-criticism often intensify. The discrepancy between others' happiness and your inner desolation can be agonizing.

The Christmas and Hanukkah season may become even more unbearable because of its overwhelming emphasis on children and the high visibility of family togetherness. Children are everywhere. Watching a youngster sitting on Santa's lap is poignant—the child is not yours. Hanging stockings up on the mantel only reminds you that it is still another year with but two people present.

> *Various people suggest that you hang stockings for your pets at Christmas—that it'll make you feel better. Well, I have a cat and dog whom I love dearly, and I've been hanging their stockings for years. But, somehow, it just doesn't quite make it.*

Then there is the impact of the Christian symbols that focus on the birth experience—the Madonna and Child lit up in Nativity scenes.

> *Even the post office, which generally distributes two holiday stamps each year, always has one with Madonna and Child. I couldn't bear the thought of licking all those religious "fertility" stamps for my Christmas cards, so invariably I'd pick the other stamp—even if I didn't like it. Sounds ridiculous, I'm sure, but every little reminder hurts.*

These symbols are a painful reminder of one's inability to have a child, and they intensify feelings of emptiness. Institutional religion (attending services or musical performances) also tends to be a greater part of people's lives during the holidays, complicating your feelings if you are angry at God and disillusioned by the Church for allowing such suffering. You may feel torn by the religious traditions you have always kept on holidays and your present rage over unanswered prayers.

Holidays are difficult because they mark specific occasions on which people base fantasies and hopes. It is not unusual to fantasize for months before an event, whether it is your birthday, an anniversary, or a holiday, that when that occasion arrives you will be excitedly announcing the news of your pregnancy to friends and family. Sometimes it may seem that the only way to survive a holiday is by imagining the arrival of a baby by the next time around. This deadline syndrome can bring temporary hope, but it also can result in depression when you realize that the present moment is last year's unfulfilled deadline. New Year's, for most people, is an exciting and optimistic time, but for those with infertility, it is another one of those markers that dramatically signifies an additional year of struggle and failure. It is the "by now, I certainly would have thought . . ." time that can unravel you and provide anything but hope for the coming year.

Suggestions for Surviving the Holidays

If you get significant pleasure from celebrating the holidays, then obviously these suggestions are not for you. But do keep in mind that it can be a vulnerable time. Holidays are stressful for everyone, even under the best of circumstances. Buying gifts, attending numerous social events, overeating, overdrinking, and traveling all contribute to the hectic pace everybody must endure. Coping skills that have always served you well may diminish somewhat in trying to deal with your infertility *and* cope with the normal holiday demands. Being strong does not necessarily mean that you must approach the holidays as you have always handled them. Even with the most supportive of families, the holiday season can bring great anxiety.

1. Try to think ahead about upcoming stressful times or events. Once they have arrived, it is very difficult to handle them effectively. Try to plan how best to deal with a particular event before emotional exhaustion engulfs you.

2. Eliminate the pressure placed on you that you "should" have

a wonderful time over the holidays. Recognize that you are likely to feel miserable throughout much of it and allow yourself to feel sad, rather than blaming yourself for your Scroogelike spirit. Pushing yourself to appear joyous when you feel wretched inside can lay the groundwork for holiday depression, especially if you do not allow yourself any breathers. If you happen to have a good time somewhere during the holidays, welcome the surprise and be thankful for a moment of relief!

3. Do not dwell on family traditions from your childhood and feel you must continue them. If there are traditions you enjoy, by all means observe them, but otherwise find new ways to celebrate the holidays.

Make the most of the season with your spouse. Buy special gifts for each other, choose and decorate a tree, form your own traditions as a couple. Explore other options of celebrating holidays in a childfree atmosphere. Consider spending time with friends who have no children or plan activities that are special to the two of you, like going to the theater or a favorite restaurant. Perhaps take a skiing trip or that Caribbean vacation you have been thinking about—a tan can do wonders in the middle of winter! Taking a trip is not a cure-all, but an effective way to escape holiday pressures and rekindle energies. Others may criticize you for your absence from family functions and even accuse you of selfishness, but you are the one who must bear the pain of infertility when sitting around a living room full of babies and children.

4. Try to remember that your spouse is unlikely to be experiencing the same feelings about infertility at the same moment as you. A situation you may be able to tolerate, or even are looking forward to, may be intensely difficult for your spouse. The importance of open communication with each other cannot be emphasized enough at this time.

5. Recognize that holidays may cause you to revive behaviors or feelings around the issue of infertility that you thought you had shaken off or resolved. It is normal for individuals to regress somewhat during this time.

6. Take care of yourself during the holidays. A lack of sleep, excessive drinking, or overeating are apt to increase irritability, poor self-esteem, and overall vulnerability. These problems are also likely

to impede sexual functioning, which probably is already showing signs of strain. This is a time when you may want to pamper yourself or indulge in something frivolous. Do something nice for yourself just because it feels good (buy yourself a gift, get a new hairstyle, or take a day off from work just to relax).

7. Visit others for only as long as you are feeling reasonably comfortable and enjoying the company. In social situations, the pressure of acting as if everything is okay can be enormous, so recognize that after any difficult social event you are probably going to need a rest—and you deserve it. Be selective in your participation in holiday events, and take care to keep them as free of pain as possible. For example, if the unwrapping of Christmas gifts is a stressful time, explain that you will be coming later for dinner.

8. Let others know what you are sensitive about, so that perhaps they can be more understanding and help you avoid uncomfortable situations. You will need all the support you can get.

9. Reduce the general holiday stresses, which affect everyone, by shopping early, trying not to overplan the holidays, and not driving yourself to distraction in order to find that perfect gift (which probably does not exist). Keep your entertaining as simple as possible. If you are unable to complete your shopping before the crowds descend on the stores, at least avoid shopping in the malls. They are overflowing with the people you are so sensitive to— mothers and babies, pregnant women, and children visiting Santa.

10. Be aware of your medical needs at this stressful time. Will a new treatment introduced in December provide a hopeful, calming influence or will it bring on new anxieties? Would it help to take a short break from treatment during the holidays or will this only exacerbate feelings of failure? Everyone has different needs and different reactions to infertility, so these are decisions only you can make.

11. Find personal meaning in the holidays that raises your spirits rather than deflates them. If you focus on Christmas as a celebration of birth, you set the stage for feeling angry and cheated. If, instead, you view this holiday as a time of renewal, you may find new strengths within yourself.

12. Sometimes it is helpful to focus on others who are less

fortunate than yourself and try to bring some joy to their world. An individual who is sick, elderly, or completely alone may find great pleasure in your willingness to give, and it may help you feel less ineffectual.

13. A special note regarding Mother's Day and Father's Day is necessary because these holidays can be particularly wrenching. One way to handle them is to focus on your own parents or grandparents by making it a special time for them. It will not take away the pain, but it may help to lessen it. If you attend church regularly, be aware the joys of parenthood may be emphasized in the service. Decide whether that particular morning at church will give you comfort or make the suffering worse. Sometimes a clergyman, if he is sensitive to your feelings, may be willing to share a prayer for those who yearn to be parents but have not yet been able to have children. If all of this still hits too close to home, find some other way to spend the day that will either give you pleasure or, at least, help you avoid dwelling on the emptiness inside.

14. Finally, recognize that the holidays *will* end and it is normal to feel relieved when they do!

These suggestions will not necessarily make your holidays a joyous time and eradicate the blues, but they can help make the experience a little more tolerable. I do not recommend escape or isolation as a general coping device for infertility. Holidays are notably stressful, however, and it is a time when breathers may be necessary. If you can accept the bittersweet nature of the holiday season and react to it accordingly, you have a good chance of emotionally surviving and perhaps even renewing your spirits. This is a time of suffering, but it does not have to be a time of feeling alone. Be willing to let people who care about you into your world, and the pain, at least, becomes bearable.

Advice to Friends and Family

Unless you have experienced the trauma of infertility, it is difficult to know *automatically* how to respond to someone in the midst of it. The following suggestions may provide some insight and give you concrete ways to help relate to your loved ones during this painful time.

1. Understand that handling infertility is a process. There are no quick or easy answers, and an infertile person does not resolve intense feelings overnight. Mood swings are common, and at times the feelings may be enormously painful. To complicate matters, there may be times when these individuals feel like talking and other times when they need some distance. Try to be patient—the infertile person needs your acceptance and understanding.

2. Listen to what the couple has to share—their pain, frustration, and anger—and try to imagine what they are experiencing. Avoid giving advice or trying to provide answers unless you are asked or feel that you have some crucial information. Understand that people often give unsolicited advice that reflects a lack of knowledge or sensitivity, so that the couple may already be fed up with outside intrusions. Presenting strong opinions also may set up a situation in which a couple feels a conflict of loyalty: one friend or relative says they should follow one route and another espouses a different view. Whether you realize it or not, listening can be the most helpful gift you can offer, something that is not always easy to do.

3. Share with the couple your concern and support so they know they are not alone. One friend of an infertile person offered these thoughts:

> *Infertility means gauging someone's moods and hating to say "how's it going?" because you're afraid of causing more pain. It means watching that pain in a friend you love and feeling it—maybe not in the same way, but still feeling it. It means thinking about what you say before you say it and not wanting to be the means of causing any more hurt. It also means wanting to bite your tongue off when you blow it. Most of all it means thinking of your friend often and wishing there was more you could do. It means the constant desire to be there for her, to take her into your arms and offer a shoulder to cry on, always.[1]*

Everyone experiencing infertility could use a friend like this woman.

If you are at a loss for words, say so ("I wish I knew what to say or could help in some way. Is there anything I can do?"). Otherwise, silence may be interpreted as rejection or lack of concern. Don't be reluctant to open your mouth for fear of saying the wrong thing. As long as you can convey your feelings of support and caring, most infertile people will understand an occasional tactless remark. Even though you have probably not experienced infertility, it is likely that you have struggled through some other significant loss, like the death of a loved one or a divorce. It can help to recollect your suffering and to remember what kind of help and support was most comforting to you at that time. The feelings may not be dissimilar.

4. Avoid asking the infertile woman if she is pregnant. Believe me, she will let you know if and when it happens.

5. Respect the couple's need for privacy, but let them know you're there when they might need you or want contact again. An occasional brief call or note can help you stay in touch and let them know you care.

6. Be honest in telling of your own pregnancy or that of others. As painful as the news may be to the couple, it is usually better than keeping it secret. Acknowledging their pain is the most helpful action you can take. Understand that the tears they may shed do not reflect malice, only sadness and anger at their own emptiness.

7. Be aware that reactions differ from person to person and from day to day. Understand that for some people there may be a need to isolate themselves occasionally, especially from events involving children.

> Socially, we tend to shy away from experiences where there are babies and small children present. Often, at work, I will find myself talking with a group of people and the discussion will turn to childbirth and kids. It is all I can do not to just walk away. I wonder if they notice that I don't participate. Also, my sister is pregnant right now and I have already warned her that I may not go to the hospital to see her. I don't know how I would react, and I would hate to embarrass her or myself by getting upset in public.

Please realize that when the infertile couple visits you, it may be a wrenching experience to watch you with your children. If they seem to find pleasure in contact with your children, then by all means offer it. Otherwise, do not ask them to hold or feed your baby.

8. Try not to offer false hopes ("I'm sure you'll be pregnant by the summer"). Infertile people play enough games with themselves without the additional burden of your denial. Also be careful about sharing the success stories of others.

> *I know others mean well, but it always seems that they give the same reaction—a story about someone who waited twenty-five years and got pregnant! If I hear one more miracle story, I'm going to throw up.*

9. Humor has its place in dealing with the struggle of infertility, but do not be the one to joke about it—leave that to the one experiencing it. A remark like "Sorry you're not pregnant, but it sure must be fun trying!" is not only hurtful but probably untrue. Nor should you diminish the impact of infertility by comments like "It's really not so bad. Think how much worse things could be. Did you hear about so-and-so who . . . ?"

10. Do not say directly or insinuate in any way that the couple's inability to conceive must stem from inner doubts about their desire to have children or must mean that God has not found them suitable for parenthood. Comments like these can be devastating.

11. Support the couple's decisions regarding medical treatment or resolution as best you can, even if you do not agree. They probably feel enough turmoil already without you adding your advice—unless of course they have requested it.

> *My mother was terrified by the fact that I was on infertility drugs. She just couldn't understand how I could put my body through all of this. As much as her concern only reflected love, I finally had to say, "Hey, Mom, bug off! It's something I have to do."*

> *My family still pretends our infertility doesn't exist. I would like for them to start to accept that it may not happen—we may not conceive a child. They avoid the fact that we may adopt. When I announced that I'm*

only going through a few more months of testing and treatment, they reacted as if I was a quitter. I should hang in there, they say. I really want them to be excited that we've decided to adopt.

12. Learn about infertility so that you can be an informed listener.

13. Refer a couple to an infertility support group, such as RE-SOLVE, if you feel they could benefit from education, referral, or additional support.

Infertility and the Couple

How Infertility Affects the Couple

"I feel like I'm talking to a brick wall."

"You don't care about this as much as I do."

"You know I'm exhausted—can't we wait until tomorrow?"

"If you really loved me, you'd (a) come with me to the doctor's appointment; (b) listen to me; (c) talk about this more; (d) drop the subject; (e) wear boxer shorts!"

But, the bottom line, probably not verbalized, is "If you really loved me, you'd make this all better."

Going through infertility can feel like you're going through hell. It is a frustrating and frightening time, made all the more maddening by its out-of-control nature. You want someone to understand the intensity of your pain and you want someone to make the pain go away. What better person to place these responsibilities upon than your spouse!

It is unusual for a couple *not* to feel significant stress on their marriage during the infertility crisis. You want and need your relationship to be strong, but instead mutual strengths and support often seem to dwindle. Each of you may become obsessed with your own pain and anger; rather than uniting, the two of you may attack or withdraw from each other. The effect of infertility on couples varies, but it is unlikely that the strain on the relationship can be avoided altogether. Even the most stable marriages can flounder under the pressures of infertility. And the longer the quest for a baby continues, the greater the possibility for distortion of the relationship.

Although the marital problems described in this chapter are common to all couples, fertile or infertile, they are more likely to be triggered or exacerbated by the stress of infertility. I hope that the coping skills presented here will be valuable in all aspects of your marital life and that they will be useful long after your infertility has been resolved.

Who Has the Problem?

The experience of infertility has strengthened our marriage in that we have drawn closer together as a team sharing a common difficulty. I have been shown over and over again that my husband will not blame me, although the infertility is on my side. He views it as our dilemma, not mine. And he stresses that our relationship is most important—it would be enhanced by children but does not depend on them.

It is very important to consider infertility as a matter that involves and affects the couple, not just the person with the primary medical problem. From an emotional point of view, both of you will always be affected. Infertility can strike at the person's very core; it can reawaken old conflicts regarding self-image and sexuality for both of you. Remember, too, that in a fifth of the cases, both partners share the medical problem, and it may take a while to uncover multiple contributing factors involving both spouses. So don't just assume that it's the other person's problem. Even if only one person seems to be vulnerable to the tension of infertility, it will inevitably have some impact on the spouse.

For example, Marsha and Ed had been trying unsuccessfully to conceive for two years. After thorough testing of both partners, it was discovered that Marsha had tubal blockage, but that Ed seemed to have no problem. Shattered by the news, Marsha felt intense guilt because of her belief that the scarring of her tubes might have been due to infection from use of an IUD in the years before her marriage. Compounding this guilt was her feeling that she was depriving her husband of a child. He could no longer desire her, she thought, and she began to fear he would lose interest in her, perhaps deserting her for a "less damaged" woman. Even at the best of times, she fantasized that he was remaining in the marriage only halfheartedly. Unable to deal with her anger and frustration, she began making comments about divorce, sometimes directly ("There's certainly no reason for you to stay with me") and sometimes more subtly ("I saw your old girlfriend Karen today—did you know she has three kids?"). In an effort to reassure Marsha, Ed would tell her that having children did not really matter to him and that it was not essential to his happiness. But Marsha did not believe him and persisted in her behavior. Ed, who was saddened and frustrated by the infertility, swallowed his feelings and denied their existence. Unable to effectively resolve these feelings, he threw himself into long hours at work and began withdrawing from the relationship.

The point of this story is to illustrate that infertility within a marriage *always* involves two people. Marriage is a system in which interaction between spouses is continually occurring. The stresses on one of you and the behavior that results affect the actions of your partner and the condition of the marriage. Spouses who pretend that the problem does not belong to them are only compounding the difficulties by preventing much needed communication and support, and they may be setting the stage for destructive blame, guilt, and anger. These people will also be delaying resolution because they will fail to experience their own mourning process.

> *Initially, I felt sorry for my wife because she was the one with the problem. But I later learned the hard way that she did not want or need my pity. At the same time, I began to fully grasp that I was as childless as she—no more, no less—even though I was not the one who was infertile. It was and is a simultaneous realization that I have suffered from infertility but am personally not infertile—although I may as well be because I am childless. "I am, but am not" goes through my mind a lot. I feel anger, guilt, and probably depression, too, but never at the same time as my wife!*

"What's Happening to Our Marriage?"

When infertility is first recognized and the initial feelings explode, the two of you may be greatly supportive of each other. But since infertility is rarely solved overnight, powerful reactions of anger, depression, and guilt are likely to continue, often growing in intensity. When the feelings do not abate, it is not unusual for one of you, usually the husband, to grow weary of trying to support and console the other. Withdrawal often then occurs, not because of lack of caring, but out of frustration and a sense of inadequacy. The husband may feel that nothing he does seems to make any difference. What communication had existed up to now may gradually disappear to the point where little that is constructive is shared. One man described it this way:

> *In the beginning, I understood and accepted her unhappiness. But it just never seemed to stop. The more it continued, the angrier I became. I was definitely going through my own feelings about the situation, but I didn't want to say anything and add to her misery. Even when her period was a few days late, I'd begin to get a little excited, too. "Maybe this is it!" I'd think. Yet the thoughts stayed inside me. I knew her moods were already so erratic that I didn't want to contribute to getting her hopes up any higher. Gradually, I withdrew because I didn't know what to say and I couldn't stand to watch her crying all the time.*

Many women find that their husband's presence, just his being there, can make all the difference in the world. It does not make the problems miraculously disappear and it may not dissolve the anger, but his presence often provides an unspoken comfort and support that people may have trouble asking for.

Often it is the woman who seems most distressed by the impact of infertility, partly because being a mother is the woman's traditional role in our society and partly because her self-image may be so entwined with her ability to bear children. As infertility persists, the wife may develop tunnel vision, focusing on the single goal of motherhood, whereas her husband may be able to divert his frustrated energies into his career or outside interests. He may become impatient with his wife's "obsession" with achieving pregnancy, and she may envy or resent his uncanny ability to carry on an apparently normal life.

The feelings can be so intense now that you may feel you are the only person in the world who is so miserable. Your self-absorption can keep you from noticing or acknowledging what your spouse is experiencing. Or you may notice only his limitations, his inability to meet your needs.

When researching this chapter and talking to my husband about his feelings during our own infertility experience (of which I *thought* I had been aware), I learned to my surprise how angry he had been during much of that time. He was angry at the predicament, angry at the thermometer, angry at the pressures for sex, but most of all, angry at me. He wanted me to handle it better and to start feeling happy again—which I couldn't do at the time. When I think about this discussion, two insights emerge: first, that I was too preoccupied with my own feelings to be aware of his, so that, even when we tried to talk it out, I was still focused on myself, and second, that only now, years after the crisis, does he feel free enough to speak of his anger directly and am I open enough to listen. There is no simple answer to this problem, but certainly you should try occasionally to put yourself in your spouse's shoes and reflect on his or her position. Not an easy task.

As noted earlier, you will also probably find that your anger is directed, either openly or covertly, at your partner, who is the most available target.

> *I think the main reason we were so angry with each*
> *other is that we couldn't sit down together and deal*
> *with our feelings about the infertility. It was much safer*
> *to argue about other issues. I didn't want to face it—I*
> *couldn't tolerate the idea of being anything less than*
> *perfect. By not confronting it, I could still try to create*
> *that image.*

Since it is the woman who most frequently must face invasive testing and treatment, she may feel resentment toward her husband for not sharing the burden, despite the fact that he may be equally distressed. Problems often arise when one partner, usually the woman, has taken complete responsibility for charting daily temperatures and sexual intercourse. This responsibility can then extend to her being the one who is consistently aware of the "right time" and who is always initiating sex during ovulation. She may resent her husband for not participating in this responsibility.

On the other hand, the man may be furious with his wife for telling him when he must "perform." Many men feel bombarded by demands—during the day, at work, and at night, on the home front, for sex and communication. Often, the woman is instructed by the doctor as to what to do; when she returns home, she directs her husband—"I need a semen sample for tomorrow. Here's the container." He may feel angry, embarrassed, or used. Hostility toward both his wife and the doctor can erupt, as he begins feeling like a sexual robot.

Sometimes, too, a discrepancy exists between partners as to their degree of interest in trying to produce children. Anger can arise when the husband feels his wife is obsessed with the idea of pregnancy and no longer has any regard for the marriage, or the wife feels that he is not exhibiting enough concern in trying to conceive. This is frequently a problem in remarriages; one partner already has children from the previous relationship and needs less to start a second family. The other partner, who is infertile, desperately desires to have his or her "own" children. When there are different levels of motivation to have a child, it is not unusual for the more motivated partner to begin demanding sex, and the spouse to withhold it—a powerful passive-aggressive pattern of behavior.

It is extremely important to recognize that spouses' reactions can and usually will differ and that no reaction is right or wrong. The problem is, however, that partners often want and expect their spouse to respond like them—the same intensity, the same pain, the same openness. But not only is their timing apt not to be synchronized in handling the crisis; it may also differ in approaching resolution. One man spoke of his frustration:

> *For two years, we've been fighting over the issue of adoption. At this point, my wife refuses to even discuss the possibility and seems to cling irrationally to the idea of becoming pregnant. I just want to be a father, however that happens, and have this whole miserable experience behind us. It's tough not being able to get through to her.*

Again, I want to stress the importance of open communication and the need for compromise whenever possible. Some of the suggestions in the second part of this chapter may help you handle the kind of conflict I've described.

Marital Collapse

Because infertility can take such a heavy toll on a relationship, some find themselves struggling to salvage the broken pieces of their marriage.

> *For one and a half years my husband refused to take drug treatment to attempt to increase his sperm count and once he did, he became psychologically impotent. I voluntarily stopped treatment because I thought our marriage would break up under the pressure to "perform." I now realize that it may break up anyway. In short, our conflicts were not resolved; I just capitulated.*

On occasion, the final outcome may be divorce, although this is the exception, not the rule. One divorced man described his difficult experience this way:

> *The resolution for us was (A) continuing efforts until we knew medically we couldn't succeed and (B) ending our marriage. We did it amicably and are still close friends, but I was and still am affected by infertility. I often wonder if a lot of people think I divorced my wife just because she couldn't have a baby—the answer is no. When I'm down I have to force myself to remember that there must be a reason things happen this way and that I still may become a father, although not with the woman I originally envisioned. If not, I need to try to remember that kids alone are not the key to happiness. I see my friends' kids growing up and I sometimes feel I've wasted eight years of my life. What do I have? No wife, no kids, not even much furniture.*

Stories like this are painful, but it is crucial to remember that infertility alone does not destroy a marriage. If there are weak points in a relationship (poor communication, lack of trust, power struggles) prior to an infertility diagnosis, this crisis will exacerbate the problems. Be on the lookout for serious marital difficulties during infertility treatment and seek help early on, if necessary. Some degree of conflict and upset may be expected, but be wary when continual fighting, vicious remarks, or total withdrawal becomes the normal routine.

You need to be aware of the power of infertility and the traumatic impact it can have on a relationship. Do not underestimate its force or play ostrich, shutting your eyes and hoping the pain will miraculously disappear. Maintaining a solid relationship during and after the infertility crisis often requires serious and continued effort.

Being Single and Infertile

Learning that you are infertile does not always occur only after trying to conceive during a marriage. For some, the problem becomes evident during examination for or as a result of other medical difficulties (as in the case of DES exposure). Although most of the emotional responses described in this book apply to any infertile person, whether married or single, the effect on relationships for the single individual has some unique characteristics that need to be addressed.

Not uncommonly, the single, infertile person will withdraw from relationships with the opposite sex or will maintain such contacts only on a superficial basis. The person may jump from relationship to relationship, never staying long enough to establish any degree of closeness. At the core of this behavior is a fear of rejection should the secret of infertility be revealed. Underlying the fear is a negative self-image; the person feels defective and believes that no one will want her or him. Many come to believe that procreative ability is the major desirable trait and that, without this, they are worthless as potential mates. Obviously, most people choose lifetime partners for reasons other than their ability to produce a child, but it may he hard for the single, infertile person to believe this.

Many people in this predicament worry about how they will handle any questions regarding their interest in having children and if (or how) they should share the knowledge of their infertility. Although there are no clear-cut answers to these questions, I will make a few comments that may be helpful.

First, try to remember that men and women are attracted to one another, fall in love, and commit themselves to marriage for dozens of reasons besides reproductive ability. If, by some chance, you do get involved with someone who desires you only for producing children, you're better off knowing this early in the relationship than later on. Recognize that you are much more than just reproductive organs.

Second, I see no reason why infertility needs to be discussed until long-term plans are being considered or unless the issue of children is directly addressed during a courtship period. You do not have to "admit" it on a first date or feel pressured to reveal this information before you are ready. You can wait until you feel the relationship is a strong and supportive one. If your partner asks you about your feelings about having children, you can be honest in expressing your desire to be a parent. Whether you choose to reveal your infertility would depend on the closeness of the relationship at that point. Of course, the information must be shared before marital plans are made.

When you tell your partner about your problem, realize that he or she may be shocked at first and upset by the news. Understand that those feelings are probably not dissimilar to the ones you first experienced. It takes time for anyone to assimilate the knowledge of being infertile, and you should give your partner this time. The more open you can be about the nature of your infertility and the feelings you have, the more effective communication will be between the two of you.

Remember that there are many options available now for treating infertility and that they are increasing. An intractable problem today may be successfully treated in the future.

Key Points for Coping as a Couple

1. Remember that it is normal for infertility to cause some stress in your marriage, including how you communicate, your affection, and your sexual activity.

We've disagreed greatly on our approach to infertility, and I've felt a strong resentment toward my husband because he wanted to wait initially; he wasn't particularly cooperative with certain treatments; and he

> *doesn't want to adopt. At times, I've thought we would*
> *never make it, but in other ways it has brought us*
> *closer together. We have a mutual problem and we have*
> *to talk about it. We're also vulnerable and understand,*
> *better than anyone, that we need each other's strength.*

Having problems like these does not mean that your relationship is falling apart, only that you are experiencing a difficult time that will require extra effort to resolve. Along the way, try to maintain a sense of appreciation for the strengths in your partner and your marriage.

2. If problems are developing in your relationship, do not diminish their importance or deny their existence by saying, "Once we have a baby, everything will be better again." There sometimes is a tendency to blame everything in the marriage on the absence of a child, thus avoiding a look at what is really happening to you as a couple. Children, once they arrive, rarely resolve marital problems and may actually increase stress. If difficulties in your relationship are developing, face them and deal with them before they become overwhelming.

3. Frequent and open communication is crucial.

> *Initially, when we did not talk much about our*
> *infertility, I felt that we were being pulled apart. When*
> *we did start communicating, though, a stronger bond*
> *than ever before began to develop. Although our feelings*
> *and perceptions have been very different, talking about*
> *them has helped us to understand each other more.*

Since the struggle with infertility is a process, it is necessary to share your thoughts and emotions along the way and to be continually aware of each other's desires. The treatment of infertility and the course of resolution require much decision making, and only clear discussion can ease the difficult choices. There is sometimes a tendency to maintain silence in the hope of protecting your spouse from painful feelings or events, but usually this only magnifies the pressure.

When conflict or uneasiness occurs between you, try to be aware of how this discord relates to your cycle. For example, ovulation may be an anxiety-ridden time when fights over sex are likely to occur because there is so much pressure to "hit it right." Being able to predict these jittery times is helpful.

4. Learn to accept the fact that you and your partner are different people who will probably respond to infertility in different ways. Try not to expect him or her to completely understand your emotional experience, even if that is your fantasy.

For the first couple of years, infertility pushed me away from my husband. His insensitivity, at times, made me hate him. However, recently, I've begun to come to terms with this. My husband wants a child but has a very hard time expressing his feelings and doesn't feel the same urgency I am experiencing. I've begun to realize that it is the fact that we are so different that I first fell in love with him—he's shy, I'm friendly; he's calm, I'm excitable; and so on. I'm learning to use his calmness to quiet my urgency. We still can't talk too much about it, but I've taken the first step in trying to be friends again. I also believe that our marriage is on its way to being stronger and better than ever.

5. Understand that both of you may need to talk about your infertility with others of the same sex. Be willing to talk about marital and sexual difficulties with infertile friends. It helps to know you are not the only ones with certain problems. It is easy to feel that other couples are handling this smoothly and without conflict, for it often looks that way, on the surface. But once you begin to talk, the reality becomes more apparent.

6. If possible, try to agree on a time limit for undergoing infertility treatment. There must be mutual decisions as to the extent you are willing to go and the amount of time you are willing to keep your lives in limbo. Time limits vary from couple to couple, but there must eventually be an end point to maintain sanity.

In conjunction with this, it is very important for you to periodically reevaluate your feelings and motivation in trying to have children.

I have become so wrapped up in being infertile that I can't bring myself to even think of being a parent. The

*two just somehow don't connect, or am I blocking it
out, making myself numb, protecting myself? Our
original goal of becoming parents has somehow gotten
lost and I don't know how I even feel anymore.*

*I'm becoming more and more ambivalent about
becoming a parent. When we made the decision to try
to conceive nearly three years ago, we knew the time
was right; we were ready for the commitment. Now, it's
almost as if we've lost interest, that parenthood isn't as
important as it once was. All of this waiting has
weakened our desire, rather than strengthening it.*

After years of unsuccessfully trying to conceive or carry a baby to
term, both you and your life-style will certainly have undergone
significant changes. The original intense desire to have a family may
have dissipated, and you might be continuing your efforts only because it has become a pattern. It is possible that the journey of
weathering this crisis together and perhaps surviving with new
strengths has provided a different outlook toward parenthood. On
the other hand, it may have served only to intensify the desire.
These questions cannot be answered by anyone but the two of you.

7. As difficult as it may seem, taking a vacation from treatment
may be necessary at times to rekindle spirits and renew closeness
with one another. Many of you will find this to be impossible because of the fear that you are "missing" a month and that that month
could have been "the one." If you are able to take this break, however, it may do wonders for your psyche and your relationship. As
when you leave your job for a vacation, all the problems will still be
there when you return, but your energy level and perspective may
be different.

*I didn't realize the strain on our marriage until the
doctor took me off all drugs and charts for six months.
We'd forgotten how happy we could be together. It made
a tremendous difference.*

8. Consider going for counseling as a couple if problems in
your marriage persist. As will be described in the chapter on "Surviv-

ing," counseling can help you learn how to handle the stresses of infertility and reestablish a fulfilling relationship. It is important, however, that counseling address the emotions of infertility, not just the physical problems in a sexual relationship.

We finally went for counseling and, to our surprise, it helped. It showed us that there were reasons we felt so much anger and that it was okay to be angry. Before getting help, I was afraid to share any feelings with my husband because I didn't want to hurt him. I was frightened to admit that I had no desire to make love to him. I figured he'd think that I didn't love him and it would jeopardize the marriage. He, on the other hand, didn't want to come to me and say, "If it weren't for you, I wouldn't be going through all these financial and emotional hassles. Why did I have to pick you?" Counseling gave us permission to say these things, but it also provided an understanding between us and a sense of security. It helped us put everything out in the open. I feel more secure with my husband now because I know that he's not unhappy with me—if he were, he'd tell me. I know now that if there's something wrong, neither of us will hesitate to tell the other and we'll do something about it.

Learning to Talk about Infertility

What Is Necessary for Effective Communication?

Trying to communicate with my husband has been the most stressful aspect of infertility for me. My husband chooses to withdraw when he is upset or troubled, and generally becomes engrossed in his work. I often call him "ostrich," as I sometimes get the impression that he thinks by burying his head in the sand and closing his eyes, our problem won't need to be faced so often. I feel like I'm alone with this problem because of his silence.

Clear and frequent communication is essential for emotional survival during infertility. A significant obstacle in any marital relationship, but particularly one under the pressures of infertility, is a lack of mutual understanding, and the art of being able to understand one another requires good communication skills. Unfortunately, many people do not know how to express their thoughts and feelings in an open and clear manner.

Several common obstacles to successful message-sending are (1) not being in touch with your feelings and therefore not being able to communicate them honestly (often, people use the defense of denial or else project their feelings onto others, unable to recognize them in themselves); (2) refusing to communicate (people may simply have little practice in expressing themselves or they may resort to passive-aggressive behaviors to convey their message); and (3) always being on the attack, making hostile, critical remarks. Many people, moreover, do not know how to listen effectively. They often misinterpret messages because of preconceived ideas, wishful thinking, or personal expectations. Or they are just unable to keep their mouths shut while another is talking. A combination of poor verbalization and not listening can play havoc in a relationship.

Each of you should examine how you feel about the expression of emotions and what your pattern of communication has been throughout the years: Are you a sulker? Are you explosive and irrational? Do you hide from feelings? Do you spend a lot of time blaming? It may help to consider how your parents communicate with one another and what you were taught, directly or indirectly, about relating to others. Examine both how you tend to send messages and how you listen. The following questions may help you assess your communication ability:

EVALUATING YOUR LISTENING SKILLS

1. How often do you interrupt your partner when he or she is speaking?

2. Can you give undivided attention to your partner during a conversation or do you tend to pick up a newspaper or turn on the television?

3. Once your partner has spoken, are you quick to criticize, condemn, or evaluate? Or do you ask questions, exploring the matter further?

4. Do you quickly jump to conclusions or do you check out

with your partner what he or she has just said to ensure that you've heard the message correctly?

5. Do you let your partner know that you're interested in what he or she is saying and that you have been listening carefully?

EVALUATING YOUR ABIILTY TO SEND MESSAGES

1. Are you frequently angry, sending hostile or critical messages?

2. Do you find it difficult to put your thoughts into words or feel uncomfortable expressing feelings and therefore choose to maintain silence?

3. Do you tend to tell your partner how he or she feels and thinks, rather than speaking from your own vantage point?

4. Are you long-winded, either never getting to the point or repeating it over and over again?

5. Do you always need to feel that you're "right"?

6. Do you constantly complain?

7. Do you often make statements that you don't really mean or fail to say what is actually on your mind?

8. Do you avoid serious discussion by frequently making sarcastic or flippant remarks?

The next time you're trying to have a discussion with your spouse, silently step back and pretend you are an independent observer watching the interaction. How would that observer evaluate your behavior?

Communicating during Infertility—The Vicious Circle

One common and destructive pattern that can often develop in a relationship develops something like this: The woman is devastated by her childlessness and her whole world revolves around how to have a baby. She talks (or complains or screams or cries) incessantly about the issue and wishes her husband could feel the intensity of her pain. He tries to understand and be supportive, but he seems never to do or say the right thing. He becomes increasingly frustrated, withdrawing into a state of helplessness and anger, while his wife escalates her efforts to get his total understanding. The result is often an ever-growing distance and a one-sided conversation in which no productive communication occurs.

If this sounds familiar, both of you may be frightened by the pattern that has developed but feel unable to change it. You may even begin to doubt your marriage. If you are the woman, you are probably questioning how you could have married a man who seems so remote and unavailable; if you are the man, you are most likely asking why you never before saw signs of insanity in her!

How to Break the Pattern?

Some people may have to set up a structure for communication when a deadlock like this occurs, in order to learn to communicate in a more natural, relaxed manner. This may seem artificial and rigid at first, but it can provide the necessary experience for effectively communicating.

One such process involves setting aside an hour twice a week for discussion, agreeing that nothing will interfere with this arrangement short of a dire emergency. The structure of the discussion time can be adapted to meet your own needs, but a basic arrangement might include (1) wife speaking for twenty minutes, (2) husband speaking for twenty minutes, (3) wife taking ten minutes for questioning to more clearly understand her husband's feelings and point of view, and (4) husband taking ten minutes to question his wife. Each person's opportunity to talk should be without interruption and must be an effort to express thoughts and feelings honestly. Part of the agreement must also be to try to keep tempers under control.[1]

If one of you is willing to listen but is reluctant to talk, the "twenty-minute rule" described by Merle Bombardieri may be helpful. The purpose of this agreement is to keep infertility from taking an all-consuming position in your life and eventually to break the pattern of lopsided communication. She suggests that you agree on an amount of time (from ten to thirty minutes) to be spent each evening talking about infertility. It should be structured to the point of actually setting a timer so that the limit is not abused. Setting a time limit beforehand is also good in that you have mutually decided when to end the discussion, instead of the responsibility being placed on one of you, usually the husband. Bombardieri notes that this is not a technique to use on a particularly stressful day when an important decision must be made or a disappointing test result has been received. But it may be invaluable for handling the everyday strain of infertility. Bombardieri has found that some of the positive effects of using this technique include (1) the wife tends to speak less about infertility and presents her thoughts and feelings more succinctly, (2) the husband is more willing to listen because he is assured of an end point, (3) the wife is likely to feel she finally has an audience and therefore feels more supported, (4) both may feel relieved that the other is feeling better, (5) there is now other time in the evening that the couple can spend doing or talking about something different, and (6) in all likelihood, as the wife is doing less talking about infertility, her husband will begin to do more. Bombardieri notes that, in many cases, the wife has actually been "grieving for two."[2]

In conclusion, remember that it is the *quality* of the communication that is important, not necessarily the quantity. It is possible for people to talk or yell back and forth all day long but never effectively communicate any thoughts or resolve any issues.

> *We used to be* very *angry at each other and would blame one another because of our own guilt. There was a lot of blame to mask the pain and we hurt each other tremendously. We've learned to talk, though, and work through it. We also have become aware of what we've let infertility do to us. That's the positive part—seeing what we've done and starting to talk long and hard. RESOLVE, in particular, has helped us to feel comfortable in discussing it.*

Making Decisions

Making decisions about anything can be hard, but when those decisions involve the multitude of feelings regarding infertility, the process can be excruciating. For example:

Should you change doctors?

What about AID?

Is it time to stop treatment?

Should you apply for adoption?

Is surgery the answer?

These are just a few of the difficult questions you must face during infertility. To compound matters, the decisions must involve *two* people, which means that not only do each of you have to face crucial issues within yourself but that you must establish agreement or compromise. For some, the decisions will come easily and with little question. For most, though, decision making will be a gut-wrenching experience in which conflicts between spouses easily explode.

The following are some important points to consider when you are plagued by the need to make a decision but at the same time, feel overwhelmed by marital conflict:

1. Don't panic if initial discussion brings sharp disagreement. Recognize that decision making is an anxiety-provoking experience and that it is a process. If you immediately react with withdrawal or angrily put up walls, the process can't progress. For example, say your spouse suddenly declares, "I think we should just forget the idea of having kids." You may immediately feel a sense of desperation and want to respond with rage. Instead, take a deep breath and try to calm down. You can state your own point of view ("I don't think I could live without children"), but try to listen to what your partner is saying. Talking about it does not mean you have to do it.

2. Recognize that decisions often come about gradually. People can feel differently in the beginning than they do at the end, after discussion and soul-searching have clarified the issues. For example, as will be described later in the discussion of adoption, couples often require years to reach this particular decision. Just because you are opposed to an idea at first does not mean you will always feel that way. Give yourself time—often time itself creates new understanding. Meanwhile, be willing to keep *talking, talking, talking*.

3. Gather as much information as possible on the subject of your decision. If it involves a change of doctors, for example, schedule a consultation or two with other physicians, contact RESOLVE, and speak to others who are in infertility treatment.

4. Try to be optimistic in your decision making. Infertility frequently creates such pessimism that it is easy to overwhelm yourself with destructive thoughts.

"Everything possible has gone wrong. I know whatever decision we make will be wrong too. Why shouldn't it be?"

"We're in so much conflict that we'll never find an agreement. It's hopeless."

Feelings like these, though not unusual, can interfere greatly with communicating and exploring options.

5. Each of you needs quiet time to consider the situation by yourself. The more clearly you understand yourself and your feelings, the more clearly you will be able to express them to your partner. People are often filled with ambivalence, despite the fact that what they say out loud seems rather definite. Carefully explore the personal reasons you have for feeling the way you do, and be willing to admit any inner turmoil that perhaps has been hard to face. Often, conflict between spouses arises because individuals are actually in conflict within themselves. Make a list of pros and cons before jumping into an argument with your partner.

6. Use the guidelines for "fighting fairly" at the end of this chapter to help with the problem-solving process.

7. Understand that whatever decision you make, there is always the potential for some regret. This is normal because decisions are rarely perfect. You must often give up something in order to gain something else. For example, in the midst of infertility treatment, you may decide that it is necessary to leave your job because of the intense demands of medical treatment. From a positive standpoint, this will give you more available time for doctors' appointments and less pressure in balancing conflicting schedules. On the other hand, it may mean putting a hold on your career and giving up certain pleasurable work-related activities. In examining your position, assess how strong the regrets might be for each alternative and try to determine which decision would probably bring the *least* discontent.

8. Recognize that the struggle of making a serious decision is usually the worst part of the ordeal. Chances are you will feel much better once you have reached some final determination.

The Inevitability of Conflict

All couples should learn constructive ways of managing conflict, and for those in the throes of infertility treatment, this is critical, especially if they have not developed healthy means of reconciling differences in the past. Individual resources tend to be sorely taxed at this time with sensitivities close to the surface and tensions rapidly rising. Intense anger is a common feeling during infertility, and your spouse may be the most available target for your rage and resentment.

> *I was basically very angry with myself and realized after awhile that I was developing all kinds of self-punishing behavior. I also gave my husband reason to punish me through anger by purposely forgetting to do something or constantly nitpicking. I really felt that someone should be angry with me.*

On the other hand, some people who are very uncomfortable with their anger and try to deny, rationalize, or suppress those feelings, rather than initiate any conflict. In either event, when discord is present, it is impossible to avoid it forever, so it is advantageous to learn some constructive means of dealing with it.

Conflict between spouses is natural, normal, and inevitable, and in itself will not damage a relationship. Without it, in fact, a marriage may become apathetic and unsatisfying. As the book *Marital Love and Hate* puts it:

> *Spouses usually are not malicious because they are out to wipe us off the face of the earth. For the most part, our spouses' anger springs from the anxiety that is inevitable in all human beings as we all are forced to search for the strength with which to live our troubled lives. In that sense, we should seek to reconcile ourselves to some outbursts of our partners as inevitable, and so too our own, as we both express our humanness and limitations.*[3]

How Conflict Presents Itself

Sometimes the conflict regarding infertility is direct and clear-cut— the issues are obvious. Most people, though, at first find it very difficult to directly confront their feelings. Trivial arguments often develop as a displaced reaction to the more serious issues of being infertile. It is likely to sound like this:

> *There were times when I just felt like picking a fight all month long and eventually that's exactly what happened. I would get upset and provoke an argument about anything; my husband was the same way. I could come home and clean the house, wash and iron the clothes, make dinner, and John wouldn't say, "Gee, honey, you got a lot done today." Instead, he'd snap, "You left the ironing board up." I would look at him and say, "Why did you get home so late?" "Why didn't you call me today?" or "You forgot to take out the garbage!" Things that normally didn't bother me became major issues. It took awhile to recognize that the underlying problem was our infertility—that we felt we were failing ourselves and each other.*

When important issues are camouflaged this way, the listener must be sensitive in order to break through the concealment and clarify the real problem. Sometimes a small irritation can serve as a re-minder of a more intense issue and can easily spark conflict that on the surface seems to be all out of proportion to the annoyance. Learning to interpret the many signals your spouse transmits is im-portant in handling differences. For example, a woman may com-plain about her husband's excessively long work hours and lack of attention to home when actually she is feeling self-critical because of her infertility and is questioning whether her husband still loves and desires her.

On other occasions, a fight may break out solely for the purpose of blowing off steam. Infertility is full of infuriating circumstances! Recognize when your partner only needs an opportunity to vent some hostility and pent-up pressure. Perhaps a woman spent a hec-tic, frustrating day balancing various medical appointments and sit-ting long hours in doctors' offices. On arriving home, she starts to rant and rave about a minuscule irritation. A sensitive and smart spouse will let her explode and wait for her to simmer down, rather than getting caught up in the details of the minor irritation.

Each partner has responsibilities in the event of a conflict—

whether it is direct or indirect. Be aware of your own feelings when provoking a fight, and if you are on the receiving end, try to evaluate what is happening. Sometimes a direct question can quickly clarify the situation ("Are you angry at me for some reason or did you just have a rotten day?"). Depending on your assessment, you can either confront the situation head-on or try to moderate it to avoid a battle.

Sources of Conflict

Conflict during the midst of infertility can result from a variety of causes:

1. Disappointment in your spouse; the feeling that he or she is imperfect: No one can be everything another person needs or wants, so there are bound to be times of anger, resentment, and hatred for the shortcomings you observe in your spouse. As McCary notes in his book *Freedom and Growth in Marriage*:

> *The more a person is unable to accept his own weaknesses and inadequacies, the more he is apt to be self-righteously indignant when he is disappointed. The mature, realistic person knows that disappointment is inevitable in a relationship and is able to deal with it in a more straightforward manner, without taking on the additional pain of feeling morally injured. To be sure, disappointment in a loved one is painful and it arouses feelings of hatred and rage, but disappointment need not be devastating.*[4]

2. The needs and desires of one spouse clashing with those of the other:

> *Initially, we fought all the time. I kept looking for new treatments/tests, but my husband seemed uninterested and only went at my insistence. He probably distanced himself emotionally because of guilt. When I would get severely depressed, he sometimes made more attempts to get involved, but they were superficial. He showed no interest in new advances, so I finally gave up and put all my energy into adoption. Once our energy was*

*directed away from infertility and toward adoption, our
relationship improved immensely and now I feel we are
stronger after having gone through all of this. My
husband has finally become supportive and interested
in our adoption pursuit, with the prospects being more
positive and tangible. Both of us feel comfortable with
our decision.*

Recognize that in facing conflict during infertility that there is
rarely a right or wrong point of view—it is strictly a matter of
opinion or individual need. As hard as it may be, attempt to understand your partner's position. Try stepping in his or her shoes for a
while. Just because you listen and try to grasp what your partner is
saying does not mean that you have to agree. It only means that you
accept the fact that you have different opinions.

Understanding each other doesn't ensure that a solution will be
reached, but it does set the stage for constructive communication so
that you may eventually find agreement or compromise. As you are
talking, watch for any points where you are in accord, rather than
just focusing on the conflict.

3. The assumption that your spouse perceives everything in the
same manner that you do: Accept the fact that no two people feel
and think in exactly the same way. Couples who approach marriage
expecting always to have identical opinions and needs are in for a
rude awakening and a rough journey. Individuals enter into marriage
with different family and social backgrounds encompassing intricate
value systems. To complicate matters, each individual carries specific
biological characteristics and personality traits. Two people simply
cannot be carbon copies of each other, always needing and wanting
the same thing.

*I'll never forget the experience of going to our first
RESOLVE meeting. My husband wasn't too excited about
the idea—in fact, that's a gross understatement—but
was willing to accompany me. I was nervous and
questioned whether it was worth the trouble of going.
We ended up fighting the entire way there and almost
turned around several times. After my anxiety lessened,
I found that the meeting was very informative and*

> *enjoyable. I commented about this to my husband on the way out and told him how much I was looking forward to other meetings. His reaction was clearly not the same. He didn't find it particularly helpful and couldn't see much value in continuing. I was furious and failed to understand why he wasn't as excited as I was. We later attended more meetings but only after accepting each other's position. I needed to understand that this wasn't the way that he was most comfortable in handling our infertility, and he had to understand that I needed the security and caring of his presence at the meetings.*

Try to develop insight into your spouse's point of view so you can better understand and anticipate his or her reactions. The ability to predict each other's behavior can help moderate the tension and instability that arises from infertility.

4. One or both of you are experiencing an internal struggle: When people are torn by inner conflicts, they are less able to handle discord between themselves effectively. A woman may be worrying, for example, about her sexuality and her sexual relationship with her husband. She knows the importance of following the doctor's instructions about intercourse but has little interest in having sex. Although she wants her husband to show her he still desires her physically, she may set up rejection because of her own negative feelings about her sexuality. Her need for control over her cycle and the pattern of intercourse may clash with her feeling that her husband should be taking more responsibility so that she may lean on him. If she cannot acknowledge these conflicting needs, it is likely that she will be antagonistic toward her husband and certainly will convey contradictory messages.

If you can honestly explore your feelings, identifying your own conflicts, you will handle interpersonal conflict more satisfactorily.

Guidelines for Fighting Fairly

How a couple deals with tension and differences in marriage is crucial. Differences can lead to growth, intimacy, and sharing or they can lead to disaster. McCary notes two kinds of quarrels found in marriages:

1. *Destructive quarreling*: "concentrates on the egos of the combatants and is belittling and punishing and alienating."

2. *Productive quarreling*: "directed at the issues on which the couple differ and avoids the sensitive spots of each individual."[5]

It is obvious which kind of quarreling will have a positive effect on a marriage, but if you are feeling angry and irrational, it is easy to slip into the destructive pattern.

Here are some guidelines for helping you fight in a fair and productive manner:

1. Both of you have a responsibility to state what is troubling you—how you see the problem and how you want the relationship to change. Withdrawal ("What's wrong?" "Nothing") is both unproductive and unfair: you are asking your partner to read your mind. What I call the "crystal ball syndrome" can cut off any opportunity for communication and problem solving from the start.

> *My response to infertility was a sense of devastation, feeling that one of the most important dreams of my life had been shattered. I kept that to myself, though. I expected my husband to intuitively know how I felt. But he didn't. He acted as if it was no big deal. He was always sure that it would "work out." In my mind, I translated that attitude to mean he just didn't care or feel the way I did about having children. I was wrong—it hurt him, too. We just needed time to learn how to communicate on the issue.*

2. Focus on only one difficulty at a time. Trying to tackle multiple issues can be confusing and overwhelming. Sidetracking can also quickly escalate into a full-scale battle in which all the difficulties in the relationship, past and present, are raised and nothing is solved. For example, if you are upset because you feel your husband is not showing enough concern about the infertility problem and all the responsibility is falling on your shoulders, stick to that issue. Do not suddenly complain that he never helps around the house and leaves you with all the work.

3. If conflict seems to pervade every aspect of your life, choose a minor issue to start, rather than jump to a problem that can make

or break your marriage. Conflict resolution takes practice, so it helps to begin with more easily attainable goals.

4. Try to begin with a positive remark. For example, if you were the woman in the second guideline, you might say, "I know this past year has been very hard on you and you've done a good job of putting up with all my tirades. I appreciate your patience. However, I need to feel that we're *sharing* the responsibility for our infertility problem, and sometimes I feel like it's all on my shoulders." Let your partner know that your complaint concerns only one aspect of his or her behavior and that you are not condemning the person altogether. When you begin with something positive, your partner is more likely to listen and want to join in the mutual problem solving.

5. Be specific when you describe the issue and keep it brief—long-winded explanations are apt to fall on deaf ears. A common obstacle to successful problem solving is that the problem is vaguely defined ("You don't seem to care about anything that's going on around here") or is described in such an all-encompassing manner it is impossible to know what the specific difficulty might be ("My whole life seems to be a failure").

6. Present the problem from your own vantage point, instead of criticizing your partner's behavior. For example: "I spend miserable hours each month sitting in the doctor's office, taking my temperature, reviewing my cycle, and getting shots. It's all so frustrating and overwhelming for me." This is much better than yelling, "You don't have to do anything and don't seem to care what I'm going through."

7. Focus on confronting the problem, not assaulting your partner. Infertility is a time of great vulnerability, and it can be very destructive to make hostile, below-the-belt, personal attacks. Try to get your anger under control *before* you address the issue. If hostility rises while you are in the middle of a discussion, ask yourself, "Why am I so mad?" and "What's happening between us right now?"

8. Each partner should paraphrase what the other has already said. This allows both of you to know if the other person has understood and helps prevent miscommunication. An argument structured in this manner could go like this: the husband presents his complaint and his wife listens without interrupting. When he finishes, she re-

peats the issue, in her own words, as her husband sees it until he is satisfied she understands. She then presents her point of view while her husband listens, and he repeats her view of the issue to his wife's satisfaction.[6] Often, by handling conflict in this manner, two people can become aware that they agree more than they thought they did. The exercise also helps people think more clearly about what they are trying to relay and encourages them to listen to the message, not just feel emotional reactions.

9. After reaching a mutual understanding of the problem, further discussion should concentrate on solutions. But remember that you must have a clear definition of the problem before you proceed, or the two of you may be arguing from different premises.

Sometimes it is helpful in problem-solving to use a technique called brainstorming. Using your imagination, you think up as many ideas as possible for a solution, regardless of their apparent usefulness. A little humor injected at this point can help to ease the tension. Once all your ideas are out on the table, the two of you can pare down the list until only reasonable solutions remain, and you can explore the advantages and disadvantages of each. Solutions to problems fall into three categories: (a) consensus: a solution that both of you consider to be satisfactory; (b) compromise: a solution that involves give-and-take, wherein each of you achieves part of your goal but also forfeits part; and (c) concession: a solution in which one of you relinquishes your position and your demands in order to terminate the fight.

10. Beware of the insidious control battle, or power struggle. This occurs when partners are adamant about their positions, refusing to move an inch or to try to understand the other's point of view. Often, the specifics of the disagreement are of less importance than the need of each to be "right" and to maintain control.

If you become aware of this happening, it is important first to realize how defeating such a battle is—no one wins; in fact, both lose. Second, ask yourself why you are holding on so tightly to your own point of view, so that you refuse even to listen to your spouse's perspective. Does it, for example, represent a threat to your self-esteem? Or do you see it as a further infringement on your sense of self-control, which is already sorely taxed by the infertility experience? Finally, be willing to take a step back and modify your own position for the sake of communication. Ask questions, listen, and paraphrase what your partner has said. Once a dialogue begins, there is at least some hope for understanding—without it, all is lost.

11. It is unfair to withdraw angrily in the middle of a conflict. You do not always have to work out a concrete solution to the problem at the time of an argument (you may decide you both need to think about the issue more thoroughly and discuss it again later), but your thoughts and feelings now need to be shared. Let your partner know when you are starting to feel better, and be aware of signals from your spouse that it is time for reconciliation.

12. Remember that infertility is a problem you are experiencing as a couple, not just as individuals, and that it is important that you face the difficulty as a team, not as adversaries. *Blaming* is one of the most malignant characteristics of marital conflict and will quickly block any possibility of resolution. If you find yourself constantly putting the blame on your spouse, you might as well forget the idea of communication.

Understanding and coping with the stresses of infertility on a marriage do not come without a considerable amount of effort. It means struggling to communicate effectively and being willing to see an issue from your partner's point of view—a difficult accomplishment. Once they have achieved it, however, couples frequently report that the experience of infertility has strengthened their relationship and given them new awareness.

We were married eight years before we ever tried to have children. The six years of infertility treatment, though, caused me to view my husband and myself in new ways. On the one hand, I learned that he would "stand by me in thick and thin" and that was very reassuring. On the other hand, I learned that he, often described as a "brilliant lawyer," could be extraordinarily passive regarding infertility treatment. It was I, always the "less bright and less capable" of the pair, who had to challenge the doctors and see them wrong. It became a strength I never realized I had.

Infertility can not only create more closeness in your marriage; it can also foster individual growth. This is not to say that miserable moments of fear, silence, or anger will be absent altogether; nevertheless, surviving an infertility crisis can bring new and lasting coping skills—open communication, the capacity for conflict resolution, emotional sharing and support, and the ability to make difficult marital decisions. Sharing pain and enduring the pressures together can be a solid bonding experience that contributes to greater awareness for each of you.

> *Infertility has definitely made us closer and more appreciative of the strong bond we have together. It's been a difficult time, but we both badly wanted a child and the trauma brought out to the surface an even greater love for each other. We share the pain of the loss of "our children" and now work together to enrich our lives in other ways. Patience, prayer, talking, and listening always brought us to a decision we could both live with. We've become best friends.*

Infertility and Sex

Our sex life is definitely the hardest problem to cope with during infertility—the lack of spontaneity, the pressure, the rules. I always find myself watching the clock out of the corner of my eye and thinking, "Oh, my goodness, he's taking fifteen minutes. I wish he would hurry up!"

I think that infertility has brought my husband and me closer, except for sex. Last year we decided together to take a vacation from treatment to allow our sex life to become normal again. I don't think, though, that sex will ever be the same for us again. It has become mechanical and goal oriented, and neither of us is certain as to how we might change it.

Sex can become one of the most damaged aspects of your relationship as a result of infertility. Just at the time when you are probably feeling the need for greater closeness with your spouse, the demands of trying to conceive interfere with the pleasure of your physical relationship. The intimacy and enjoyment of sex could help you escape the strain of infertility, but sex serves only as a reminder of the pain. It becomes a revolving door: you end up feeling anxious and frustrated, which is how you felt when you started.

I was devastated when my period arrived each month. But, in a way, it was a relief because it then meant that I had ten days of freedom from sex, ten days of a celibate existence.

Rather than being motivated by passion or a desire for closeness, sex becomes ruled by the calendar and the basal thermometer reading. All the physical and emotional demands made on you during evaluation and treatment begin to have a sharp impact on your life in the bedroom. Unfortunately, anxiety, depression, and fatigue—all associated with infertility—have adverse effects on sexual desire.

Infertility does not always have a negative influence on a couple's sexual relationship; in fact, some couples report becoming closer and more intimate through sharing the stresses. The majority of people, however, will not find this to be the case, and those who do will achieve this closeness only after working through all the strains. Sex, for most of you, will become an onerous, mechanical chore, the antithesis of what you see on soap operas or read in the latest best-selling romance. Spontaneity and sensuality will in all likelihood be lost, and you may fear that they will never be recovered. Even worse can be the guilt that follows for not experiencing a loving sexual union.

Sex on Schedule

Sexual problems for most infertile couples develop because sex has become only a means of reproduction, and the emotional expression of the sexual relationship—the tenderness, the passion, the joy—is lost. Although reproduction and sexuality are not the same, society often equates them, so that the inability to reproduce is a negative reflection on a person's sexuality.

When your fertility is first being evaluated, many of you will find that your interest in sex and capacity for orgasm will dissipate.

> *With infertility, there's just too much thought when it comes to sex. Instead of being guided by feelings, everything is thought out: What day is it? Has my temperature risen? Are we in the right physical position to make love? Have I stayed on my back long enough to let those little suckers swim up inside me? At times, it would be easier to just go to a doctor's office and be artificially inseminated than to endure the experience of intercourse. It no longer seems like making love.*

All this unfortunately can increase your feelings of being damaged or undesirable. Some of you may even feel that you do not deserve an enjoyable love life because you are unable to conceive.

Keeping daily charts and scrutinizing the monthly cycle can make it seem that only the mid-cycle days of ovulation are really important. Performance pressures on the man, in particular, can become enormous and he may increasingly feel like a failure. He may also feel that his wife has no interest in him as a person, only in his sperm and his ability to impregnate her. Many of you may begin to fantasize that your sex life no longer belongs to just the two of you, but that it is you, your spouse, and the doctor all in bed together. So many intimate details of your sex life have probably been revealed that making love is not an event experienced behind closed doors. Some women may even develop the fantasies of their doctor impregnating them.

Try to remember that the temperature chart provides only a crude estimation of your cycle and that it is unwise to plan your entire life around such an inaccurate measure. I realize, of course, that this is *much* easier said than done. When daily temperature readings and maintenance of a chart become an onerous chore, many find it helpful to share this responsibility in some way (the woman takes her temperature and her husband records it; the husband takes his wife's temperature and keeps the chart; or the chart is placed in a visible spot where both can interpret it and share responsibility for initiating sexual relations).

Physicians' recommendations regarding the timing of intercourse differ, but whatever it is, most people try to follow it precisely. Despite being advised not to try to adhere to a particular regimen too closely, many people do exactly that. Often, it can be a tactical stratagem: "Well, last month we had sex on days 11 and 13; let's try 12 and 14 this month and see what happens."

Many people go to extraordinary lengths to ensure intercourse at the "right" time. One woman told of her flights to various cities around the country where her husband was attending business meetings in order "not to lose a month." Any of the following incidents might occur in an ordinary month: planning time in a busy schedule for masturbation so that the semen can be used for an insemination; struggling at midnight to have sex when you can barely keep your eyes open; or planning sex to coordinate with a scheduled postcoital test.

You can also become so exhausted by your efforts and so uninterested in making love that you sometimes forgo scheduled sex and then give false information on your monthly charts.

> *There were times that I'd get ready for a visit to my gynecologist and would review my chart ahead of time, as I knew my doctor would. Although we always had sex at least once midmonth, I was too tired and couldn't have cared less the rest of the time. It would sometimes strike me that there weren't enough X's (for intercourse) on my chart and I would imagine the doctor thinking, "Well, they sure don't have much of a sex life." So I would pencil a few more in—just for good measure.*

In trying to cope with the pressures of scheduled sex, couples often play games with each other as a means of avoiding intercourse.

> *We used to have kind of a silent joke on nights when it was clear we should be having sex. Both of us would actually stall: "Gee, I really just want to read this last thing in the paper" or "There's a great movie I wanted to watch tonight on TV—it'll be over at 1:45." We'd delay, hoping the other person would get very tired and fall asleep.*

Sometimes, partners use the results of games like these as ammunition for expressing their anger and projecting their conflicting feelings about having to make love when they don't feel like it ("I can't believe you fell asleep last night. We were supposed to have sex and you ruined it!"). Other avoidance tactics include doing household tasks or office work late into the night, complaining all the while about how much you have to do; provoking a fight just before it's time to go to bed; or suddenly thinking about all the things your partner does that aggravate you.

As you are going through infertility treatment, try to remember that making love is not just having intercourse and is not solely a matter of reproduction. Engaging in a variety of pleasurable acts—cuddling, massaging one another, having oral sex, taking showers together, varying your positions—can make scheduled intercourse less mechanical. And do not expect spontaneous arousal to occur all the time, or even most of the time, during the infertility experience. That's the unfortunate reality. You might try to be more seductive with your partner in order to encourage greater sexual interest, but, of course, that's difficult when you're feeling angry and depressed.

Avoiding the "Shoulds"

It is common for all people, not just infertility patients, to question their sex lives and imagine how they stack up against the "normal" population with regard to frequency, variety, and degree of pleasure. When experiencing infertility, however, this sensitivity to your own sex life as compared with others is apt to intensify, and feelings of being abnormal can easily develop.

> *I had always questioned whether my sex drive was lower than most people. It's not that I didn't enjoy sex—only that I didn't need it that often. Before infertility, these questions were only fleeting thoughts, but once infertility treatment began, it became a major issue for me. Sometimes I thought there must be something wrong with me. To make matters worse, I began to dread sex because of the required routine.*

It is important to find your own level of comfort and satisfaction with regard to frequency of sex. Around the time of ovulation, it may be necessary to follow the doctor's instructions and sometimes just "go through the motions," but during the rest of the month you should not put pressure on yourself. There is no right amount of sex—only that which is pleasurable for you.

With regard to frequency of sex during the middle of the month, the answer is still not clear. Some of you may feel compelled to have intercourse every day, while others of you may decide to refrain for a few days prior to ovulation to "save up sperm." For men who are fertile, no physiological benefit has been found in delaying ejaculation beyond twenty-four to forty-eight hours in order to produce more sperm.[1] And, in these men, one study has indicated that more frequent sex brings a greater likelihood of conception.[2] This is true, in part, because it increases the chances of hitting the right time. Moreover, if you have an active sex life, it probably means that you find pleasure in it and are less plagued by anxiety. In men with lower sperm counts, however, daily sex may be contraindicated because of the longer time it takes to store up sperm.

Sexual Acting-Out

On occasion, a few people may resort to sexual acting-out if the damage to their self-image has been great. Promiscuous behavior or having an affair can be an effort to repair negative feelings about oneself, to reaffirm a sense of desirability and attractiveness. This kind of behavior, however, is not common, especially if other positive aspects of the relationship (sharing interests, actively communicating, being affectionate) are maintained.

When Previous Sexual Problems Get Worse

If a couple has always had a satisfying sex life, this part of the relationship can easily suffer during the stress of infertility treatment. If sexual difficulties already exist, however, there can really be trouble as these tend to worsen under the new stress. Ask yourself if the problems you are now experiencing—impotence, premature ejaculation, lack of sexual interest, or an inability to have orgasms—began with the onset of infertility or if, to some degree, they were present before. The answer to this question can help you assess what the causes are and can suggest some solutions.

Unfortunately, those who do not already have a solid base of open communication, trust, and sexual enjoyment must work to develop it at a time when the pressures from infertility are immense. To make matters worse, many people still find it difficult to talk about sex.

It may help, in approaching the problem, to consider some of the more common causes of sexual problems. First is ignorance: many people don't know much about sex. Although the media are preoccupied with the subject and our society is thought to be sexually free, a great number of people know little about sexual pleasuring, including techniques of foreplay and stimulation. If this applies to you, do some reading. Many sexual guides are available today that provide clear, "how to" information (see Bibliography).

Another frequent cause of sexual problems is a lack of communication between partners—both an inability to express their needs and an inability to express feelings of endearment during sexual contact. Being able to openly communicate requires a sense of trust in your partner, unfearful of rejection or humiliation, and a sense of confidence in yourself, unashamed of your sexual wants and needs.

Unresolved anger also might adversely affect a sexual relationship. Women, in particular, have difficulty in expressing anger directly. The anger then is often translated into a lack of sexual interest. If a woman is chronically angry with or resentful of her partner and feels helpless to change matters by communicating her feelings, sexual desire may easily disappear.

Fear is another obstacle to sexual fulfillment. This is particularly common in men who worry that they will be unable to achieve or hold an erection. And women, too, may fear that they will fail to please their partner. In both cases, the fears derive from feelings of inadequacy and low self-esteem. If these feelings have always existed, they will surely be exacerbated by the infertility diagnosis.

Many sexual problems stem from unconscious anxiety or guilt that had its origin in childhood experiences. Sex for many is still associated with sinful behavior and carries unconscious expectations of punishment. Many adults who experience sexual difficulties were reared in restrictive homes with strict and highly moralistic parents. Their fears may make these people unable to lose themselves emotionally in the passion of sex.

Any of these causes—as well as many others—might impinge on a sexual relationship. You may have always known that sex was a problem for you but were able to avoid dealing with it. Now that infertility has struck, however, it's probably hard to ignore. Chances are that the problems have gotten worse and are therefore more noticeable. And, too, sex is such an integral part of infertility that it's impossible not to face the issues directly.

The crisis, despite its misery, can become the springboard you need to improve your sexual relationship. There is not space here to examine thoroughly all the sexual problems that might exist but I will discuss three of the more common problems experienced with infertility. Also consult the books listed in the Bibliography for specific advice. Lonnie Barbach's *For Each Other* may be especially useful in providing exercises for enhancing both the physical and the emotional aspects of your sexual relationship.

Struggling with Impotence

Impotence refers to the inability to maintain an erection, thus preventing sexual intercourse from taking place. It can be caused by psychological or physical factors, although the first is the more common reason among younger men. Often it is only temporary and is related to fatigue and stress. Men normally will experience impotence at some point in their life (statistics indicate an 80 percent chance of its occurring).[3] During infertility, however, it becomes especially likely because of the stress during evaluation and treatment and the negative impact on self-esteem. "Sex on command," too, can be extremely difficult to manage.

One of the most common times for temporary impotence to occur is when a postcoital test is scheduled. The necessity of having intercourse a certain number of hours before a doctor's appointment certainly qualifies as a pressure-cooker situation. It is hoped that most physicians will be understanding about the emotional impact of this arrangement and be willing to make alternative plans should impotence occur. Some men also experience impotence when they need to produce a semen specimen for evaluation. The pressure is usually less on this occasion because the woman need not participate and timing may not be as critical. There are situations, however, when ejaculation must occur in the physician's office and that can be nerve-wracking. Not only stress but fatigue, alcohol, and certain medications can also contribute to impotence.

Men are not likely to discuss this problem with their peers, so they may well feel alone and threatened by its occurrence.

When impotence first happened to me, it was a complete shock. It made me feel like a failure. I couldn't understand why my body wasn't working like it should. To my wife, I made an excuse and pretended like it was no big deal, but inside I was frightened. Having infertility problems was bad enough, but to compound that with impotence was just too much to handle.

A man with this problem may be reassured to know that impotence, under these circumstances, is usually temporary and relief from the pressure of "performing" can renew erections. If his self-image is strong, he will probably take this temporary problem in stride but if he is already feeling inadequate, the difficulty may seem to him just further evidence of his failure. The pressure to perform and the fear of failure can then become self-perpetuating.

It is very important for the woman to be aware of her own reactions to impotence.

When my husband briefly experienced impotence, it was probably as bad for me as it was for him. With all the other worries we had, that one caught me totally by surprise. I immediately jumped to the conclusion that it was happening because he was no longer attracted to me. I felt I must be doing something terribly wrong.

Women commonly ascribe blame to the problem of impotence, failing to recognize that the condition is out of the man's control. Since the woman may have had to face extensive testing and treatment herself, she may directly or indirectly be giving her husband the message that he better "keep up his side of the deal." This pressure, or any kind of confrontation that seeks to get to the bottom of the matter, is likely to be counterproductive at this early point. If the situation is occurring for the first time, it is probably best not even to push for a discussion. That may just make an issue out of something that is really not a problem. If the difficulty continues and it seems likely that stress is causing it, try to be understanding and encourage your husband to share his worries. Also let him know that you still find him desirable. When depression exists, determine whether impotence has led to these feelings or vice versa.

If the problem persists, a complete physical examination would be in order to determine if there are any physical causes. Sexual counseling may also become necessary. The usual approach is to discontinue intercourse for a period of time with instruction to focus on sexual pleasuring experiences—touching, holding, fondling, massaging—and to restore the capacity to relax. Masters and Johnson refer to these exercises for beginning to think and feel sensually as "sensate focus."[4] The American Medical Association Committee on Human Sexuality states: "Because most impotence is a maladaptive reaction, the treatment is one of unlearning, not learning. Treatment is specifically directed at removing the man's fear of failure, the wife's fear concerning the man's performance, and the man's desperate attempts to will his own actions."[5] When impotence does occur, an intensification of attempts at intercourse may be the worst possible response because it is only likely to aggravate the problem.

Dealing with Premature Ejaculation

Premature ejaculation is another condition that can already exist prior to the infertility diagnosis or can result from the anxiety of infertility treatment. It is probably the most commonly experienced sexual problem for men and is usually psychogenic in origin. Because of the pressure for ejaculation to occur within the vagina during infertility treatment, premature ejaculation prior to penetration can be a humiliating and frustrating experience.

In treating this problem the wife is often involved in the therapy and is taught ways to assist her husband. It is important that she not become impatient and resentful because her willing participation in overcoming the difficulty is necessary. One very successful technique that is frequently used is the "squeeze technique."[6] This involves stimulating the penis until ejaculation is just about to occur. At this point, the man's partner squeezes the glans of the penis for about ten seconds, causing dissipation of the urge to ejaculate. Sometimes the man needs only to tell his partner to stop stimulation when close to orgasm, proceeding again when his erection has gone down. This technique helps the man develop greater control during stimulation by concentrating on the sexual sensation and on the ability to regulate it. Based on the work of Masters and Johnson, the success rate in treating this condition is 97.8 percent.[7]

Lack of Sexual Interest

The biggest problem for me was an absolute lack of desire. There was a lot of fantasizing. I'd rather have been with anyone, including the milkman, than face sexual relations with my husband. It became boring, pressured, and so unspontaneous. It was like watching "Playboy Channel" every night on TV—it just became repetitious. Plus the pressure to have to perform on certain nights was so uncomfortable. On Monday, I

might feel like it, but knew that Tuesday was really the
"right" night. Then, on Tuesday, I could be nauseous
and vomiting, but we had to have sex. It all became
too predictable. I lived in Florida for many years and
sex became like the weather there. As pleasant as it is,
you hate it after awhile because you always know what
to expect. I had it down to a science—I could tell
whether sex was going to be a 1, 2, or 3, with 1 being
the best, which meant a lot of foreplay and caressing; 2
was okay, better than a quickie; and 3 meant "wham,
bam, thank you, ma'am." Often times, though, the best
for me was a 3 because that's all I wanted to do.

Like other sexual difficulties, lack of sexual interest may be a long-standing problem or one that has developed since the onset of infertility. Routine sex and monthly disappointment can unquestionably in themselves diminish sexual desire. The only exception might be at time of ovulation. But making love even then can take on an overtone of "I don't really feel like it, but it's the right time." Relationships often develop a platonic feeling, a sense of deep closeness, through the suffering that is shared, but sexual feeling may well be lacking.

A major difference, however, in the impact of men's and women's sexual difficulties is that intercourse and conception can occur regardless of a woman's sexual problem (lack of desire, orgasmic difficulties), whereas the husband has more at stake. He knows that his sexual difficulty, especially if it is impotence or premature ejaculation, may be preventing conception, and thus he is under greater pressure. The woman's problems, too, are usually not obvious and can be less of an issue between partners. Of course, that does not mean that the woman is less disturbed by her situation.

Contributing factors to a lack of sexual desire are many. It is important to determine when the problem began so you can assess its causes. Those who have never or rarely had any sexual interest probably had childhood experiences that severely affected their sexual functioning. This could include incestuous experiences, rape, or repressive sexual teaching from parents or religious figures.

More commonly, in infertility, the problem occurs among women who once enjoyed sex but have lost the desire or women who have only sporadic interest. Depression, anger, and guilt—

common during the infertility experience—can negatively affect sexual desire. And the fatigue from pursuing infertility treatments or balancing work and medical schedules can easily leave women physically and emotionally depleted.

Lonnie Barbach states that the most common cause of lack of sexual desire lies in the nonsexual aspects of the relationship with one's partner.[8] If you are angry or dissatisfied with your spouse, and are feeling powerless, you may withhold sex as a way of maintaining some control in the relationship. If feelings of anger and blame are the rule rather than the exception, it's not surprising that interest in making love diminishes. Sometimes the anger does not concern a current issue but rather an unresolved dispute from the past.

Other factors that might lessen sexual desire include fears of intimacy, a lack of physical attraction to one's partner, or a history of unsatisfying sexual experiences. The last cause may derive from inadequate knowledge about sex, so that partners are unaware of how to arouse each other. It may also stem from inadequate communication, with partners unable to express what brings them the most pleasure.

In the midst of an infertility crisis, it is difficult but not impossible to remedy the problem of low or nonexistent sexual desire. The first step is to determine when your sexual relationship *was* fulfilling and what elements made you interested in sex. Was sex more enjoyable when you were relaxed and on vacation? Were you more attracted to your partner after you had a heart-to-heart talk and felt he was more understanding? Were you turned on early in your relationship when both of you were making conscious efforts to please each other and sex was more exciting? Learning what once sparked your sexual interest will give you clues for rekindling that desire.

If unresolved anger and poor communication are the likely culprits in destroying your sex life, some of the suggestions in the chapter "Infertility and the Couple" may be helpful. When partners are able to express their hurts and dissatisfactions—both past and present—and become more sensitive to each other's feelings, they can then move on to renewing an enjoyable sex life.

If part of the problem is the routinization of sex during infertility, you may have to work consciously at creating diversity and excitement, at planning and anticipating pleasant times together. As Lonnie Barbach says:

*The myth that good sex is spontaneous grows out of
distorted memories of the initial exciting lovemaking
sessions with a partner. Of course, the novelty of a new
sexual relationship and learning about each other
creates an excitement all its own. But the spontaneity
that occurs during the early stages of the relationship
actually results from considerable attention and
planning. Dates are often made in advance, providing a
period of hours or days during which anticipation can
build. Attractive clothing and even sexy underwear are
worn and the bedroom or whole house or apartment is
often cleaned in anticipation. Then, the evening begins
with some intimate activity undisturbed by outside
intruders. Finally, somehow, at the end of the evening,
you end up in bed together, and this is considered
spontaneous.[9]*

Good sex, early or later on in a relationship, requires some effort
and preparation.

Infertility has the power to make a relationship grow old very
quickly. You and your marriage may be young, but the pressures
inherent in infertility treatment and its effects can make you feel
you've been married for many years. Most couples don't have to face
this predicament until much later in their relationship.

This means that you have to work at keeping your relationship
alive and special: find new places to make love; take extra care to
make yourself attractive and sexy; notice your partner's attractiveness; plan special times together that you can anticipate; and tell
your partner, "I love you." If you can make your sexual relationship
work during the course of infertility, one thing is certain—you will
have learned some valuable lessons for keeping your marriage strong
and vital when the crisis has passed.

Responding to a Final Diagnosis

Once a final diagnosis of infertility has been confirmed, you will
enter a period of intense mourning that also takes its toll on a sexual
relationship. Feelings of apathy toward sex or a wish to avoid it
entirely are not uncommon at this time. Even if you originally

viewed sex as a pleasurable activity in its own right, you may gradually have come to perceive it as serving only the function of reproduction. When that function is gone, an attitude can develop of "Why bother?"

In other cases, one or both of you may respond to a final diagnosis by denying your grief and overcompensating with a strong effort to prove your sexual prowess, interest, or desirability ("What's the big deal? We can still have a great sex life!"). This reaction is not likely to be effective on a long-term basis, though, and will only prolong the time until honest exploration and acceptance of feelings must take place.

Recognize that it takes time to heal after experiencing infertility.

What really gets you through sex during infertility is the continual hope of "maybe this will be the month." The real damage comes after you have resolved the problem in some way. At that point, after all we'd been through, I just didn't want to be bothered anymore. We had learned to tune each other out and that continued long after our infertility treatment was over.

As Barbara Eck Menning pointed out in her book *Infertility: A Guide for the Childless Couple*, there is usually a "moratorium on sex after the final diagnosis, corresponding roughly to the period of grief, when both the man and the woman do not wish to have relations."[10] The two of you will probably require different amounts of time to resolve your feelings, and you will need to be sensitive to each other's needs. If one of you feels prepared for renewing an active sex life but the other is not ready, masturbation may have to be the temporary solution. Or finding ways of gentle pleasuring as a couple can be a compromise step.

In any event, you will have to work at renewing your sexual relationship. You may even have to push yourself to have sex; sometimes when you get caught up in making love, the desire itself can follow. Remember that enjoying sex is often a matter of psychological concentration, so if you make a conscious effort to focus on its pleasure, rather than allowing distractions or unpleasant memories to intervene, you may find that your sexual satisfaction dramatically increases. Again, at this time, be imaginative in thinking of new places, times, and positions. The "missionary position" performed in bed prior to falling asleep can renew painful memories. As one infertility patient said:

> It takes a lot of patience and a lot of understanding, but most of all, it takes time. That's the point at which you need to be able to get away together with a bottle of wine, probably even more so than during the infertility treatment.

Returning to an active, mutually enjoyable, and spontaneous sex life, once you have experienced infertility, is not easy, but it can be done.

Surviving the
Infertility Grind

The Infertility Grind

If you have been diagnosed as infertile, chances are that "getting pregnant" has become the most important goal of your life. Nothing else matters. You wake up thinking "pregnancy," brood over it all day long, and fall asleep with the same thought. It is an obsession.

Struggling with infertility means facing a thermometer every morning and getting stuck regularly with a needle. It means poring over your chart, searching for an answer to your unattained pregnancy. It means enduring surgery and struggling not to wet your pants for regular sonograms. Most of all, it means having to confront failure month after month. The problem takes on overwhelming dimensions and swallows up your life. The sense of failure and helplessness infiltrates all aspects of your world from work to social relationships to leisure time. All this sounds melodramatic, but if you have been there, you know it is no exaggeration.

The Monthly Cycle

Life, for the infertile woman, becomes ruled by the menstrual cycle. Calendars, for her, measure only the time from period to period. She may often forget what day of the month it is, but she is always certain of the day in her cycle.

Within each cycle, there are three identifiable phases that most seem to experience, and it is important to recognize how your emotions fluctuate with these phases. First comes what I call "The Crash," which means the arrival of menstruation and the often intense feeling of loss it brings. It is a time of acute hopelessness and feelings of failure. Women often report that they cry uncontrollably when they see that first drop of blood, followed by despair and numbness. It may take several days to reemerge into the world of living.

> *The most overwhelming feeling for me occurs the day*
> *my period starts. I feel so empty, useless, and alone, and*
> *I cry for no reason or any reason. I can cope through*
> *the other days, but I hate the monthly reminder that all*
> *the time, money, and effort failed again. I want to curl*
> *up and die somewhere. How I hate that feeling, but I*
> *can't help it—I just cave in. Sometimes I have to take a*
> *tranquilizer just to balance myself out.*

Sometimes the first sight of blood is so traumatic that a woman actually denies, for a short time, that her period has arrived ("Maybe I'm really pregnant and this is just some spotting"). The pain in facing reality will eventually come, though.

Next comes the "Walking on Eggs" phase around the time of ovulation. These are days of anxiety as you take your temperature, examine your chart, and listen to the rhythm of your body, waiting to feel those twinges as an egg is released. It is also a time of sex on schedule and heightened emotions because of the pressure to do everything right.

Finally, there are the remaining days of your cycle, which I call "Fantasy Time." This stage is also marked by extreme anxiety, but this time laced with hope ("Maybe this is the month!").

> *I often let myself loose during those postovulation days*
> *and just allow my imagination to run wild with*
> *wonderful possibilities. As months and eventually years*
> *have passed, I permit myself this luxury less and less,*
> *but it always creeps in a little.*

Throughout these last days of your cycle, you will probably become keenly aware of every physical response in your body, as you wonder whether your efforts have been successful this month. Are your breasts sore and swollen? Is that nausea from pregnancy or just the wine you drank last night?

> *I feel sometimes like my body is separate from me and*

that I am playing a little game with it. I figure that "it"
knows shortly after ovulation if there is a pregnancy,
but "I" have to wait two or three lousy weeks to learn
the outcome. I search my body for clues that conception
has happened, but the signs are always so
confusing—do my painful breasts mean pregnancy or
an imminent period?

Unfortunately, some of the fertility drugs that are frequently prescribed can cause a lengthening of the menstrual cycle which only increases the tension and builds false hopes (and allows fewer cycles to occur each year). The emotional instability often felt by infertile women prior to menstruation is probably due both to hormonal changes and to the stress from the infertility process. Men, although they are not experiencing the same physiological effects, often indicate that they, too, feel increased tension at this time.

Each month takes its toll. You may rebound from the depression following menstruation and mobilize yourself again for another month's efforts, but each cycle takes a little more out of you. As one person described it, "It feels like I've been through a death each month." At some point, you may be unable to bounce back.

It helps to recognize how you fluctuate with the different phases of your cycle. When are you likely to feel most depressed or most anxious? By monitoring these emotions, you can predict your most difficult days and try to keep them hassle-free. The day you expect your period, for example, would not be the best time to have lunch with your pregnant sister-in-law. Monitoring can also help you understand why you are ready to cry at any provocation or why arguments with your spouse increase. Most important, remember that almost everyone experiencing infertility endures these mood swings—they are normal and inevitable.

The BBT Blues

I used to think, as I figured my temperature to the
nearest quarter of a tenth of a degree (a rise from
97.725 to 97.775 is at least a rise), that I'd gone right
over the edge. That was before I overheard a group of
perfectly sane, normal people discussing how to clean

*up the mercury after you throw your thermometer
across the room.*[1]

Anyone involved with infertility is familiar with the BBT, or basal body temperature. It is a sine qua non of infertility treatment—everybody has to do it. When you first begin daily charting, it can be almost fun, an intriguing study of how your body operates and of the intricacies of ovulation. But how quickly that fascination wears off!

Strangely, however, temperature taking becomes a powerful routine, probably because it is something you can *do*, even if you can't control what the thermometer says. It also has been the only readily available means of discovering what your body is doing (although new over-the-counter products for testing urine are now available). Even when the doctor tells you it is no longer necessary, you may not be able to stop. It is as though you cannot get pregnant without putting a thermometer in your mouth each morning.

Every fluctuation, no matter how minor, can bring a torrent of emotion, whether elation or depression.

> *There are times that I almost feel frightened to breathe
> in the morning, for fear that I might throw off the
> reading by a tenth. Even if I desperately need to go to
> the bathroom, that necessity always takes second place
> behind temperature taking. I sometimes lie in bed with
> the thermometer stuck in my mouth for fifteen minutes,
> one part of me irrationally praying that my
> temperature will go up further and the other part
> noting the absurdity of playing this game. If my
> temperature fails to do what I expect or want it to do,
> that fact is instantly visible—I either cry, withdraw in
> silence, or begin picking on my husband.*

Feelings about your infertility are also easily displaced onto the thermometer as the harbinger of news and symbol of frustration.

> *I invest powers in that thermometer that are clearly
> ridiculous but, after all, that little piece of glass is
> capable of making or breaking my day. For example, if
> my temperature has not gone up, it often means the
> aggravation of another trip to the doctor's for an*

insemination and that means rearranging my entire
work schedule yet another time. I have such strange
feelings toward that thermometer—I hate it, but I
need it.

Most people obviously could use a rest from this chore at some point in their infertility. But if you cannot stop and yet feel you need a break, consider sharing the charting responsibility with your spouse. Remember: the BBT chart provides only a general idea of how your cycle is progressing; torturing yourself with wishes for a "normal" chart will not help. Also keep in mind that many people who get pregnant have abnormal charts.

From a practical standpoint, many have found it helpful to use a digital thermometer, rather than the regular scaled one. Get one that displays the temperature in lighted form (it helps in early morning darkness and with fuzzy eyesight) and be sure it indicates tenths of degrees. Another advantage of digital thermometers is that they give a temperature reading accurately within one minute, which alleviates some of the anxiety of longer waits.

Torture and Torment: Tests and Treatment

Fear is an emotion I have not yet mentioned regarding infertility, and yet you will probably find it to be a familiar feeling with the onslaught of tests and treatment. It is scary to learn that you are scheduled for an endometrial biopsy, a hysterosalpingogram, or a laparoscopy—just for starters. The very words are intimidating.

Unfortunately, infertility means that you will probably have to face all manner of physical procedures being inflicted upon your body; that is just the name of the game. But somehow you do manage to get through it all. In fact, many find that procedures that terrified them the first time and that they thought they could never tolerate became almost routine.

I used to be petrified of needles. Even the blood test for
my marriage license was a traumatic event! I look back
on that time and am amazed at the change which has
happened in me—after four years of blood tests,
Pergonal shots, and probably every other treatment in

the book, it honestly doesn't bother me any more.
Getting an injection every morning is, strangely, almost
equivalent to brushing my teeth. Maybe I've just become
numb to it all. Or maybe I figure that there's nothing
more that can be done to my body that I haven't
already endured.

It has been said that infertility patients are second only to terminal cancer patients in their willingness to tolerate any kind of medical treatment.

I really feel "You can do anything that you want to my
body if you let me have a baby. I'll put up with any
amount of pain." During all this treatment, I've become
a real trooper to the point where I'm now oblivious to
the fact that my body is black and blue from injections.

That wish to have a child is powerful.

Once you have acknowledged that an upcoming test or treatment is frightening, how do you keep the anxiety from paralyzing you? The answer is to *take control* of the situation in any way you can. Let's say that you are scheduled for a laparoscopy and you have never before been admitted to a hospital. The first thing you might do is to concentrate on the event and consider what needs to be done in practical terms. If you are planning on taking off a couple days from work, you can prepare for your absence. You can also plan what you will take to the hospital with you and how your responsibilities at home will get done.

Some people find it helpful to learn about the procedure and to talk with friends about the experience. Others prefer to enter more blindly, guided by a general understanding of the operation and trust in their doctor. Although you may not want to know all the details beforehand, it is important to discuss the surgery with your doctor, including the basic technique, the necessity of the procedure, what information will be obtained, and any problems that might occur. If you have questions about the indications for surgery or any other test or treatment, do not hesitate to obtain a second opinion.

As you are anticipating the surgery, think of other stressful experiences you have successfully gone through. One helpful technique is to use positive self-talk. This means talking to yourself in a manner that helps you face stress or deal with a problem. What you say to yourself regarding an experience can have a significant effect on how you respond to it—before, during, and after an event. If your thoughts run along the lines of "I know the doctor will find something terrible," "I bet the shots will really hurt," or "What happens if I don't come out of anesthesia?" it is very easy to become panic-stricken and immobilized. Rather than working yourself into a frenzy with negative thoughts like these, try to talk positively to yourself: "Stop worrying. The surgery will go smoothly and I can get through it just fine. This information is absolutely necessary for my treatment."

It helps immensely to have the support of close friends or family in going through any difficult procedure. Do not feel that you have to be brave and face everything alone. If help is not readily offered by others, do not hesitate to ask for it. Having a spouse, parent, or good friend with you can be extremely comforting.

> *I was frightened before my first hysterosalpingogram but was reluctant to let anyone know how anxious I was. After all, I was a strong person and should be able to cope with what the doctor described as a "little discomfort." Actually, my fears were twofold: how bad was the pain actually going to be and what was the doctor going to find? I'm not sure which worry was worse, but I bottled them up inside and even told my husband that it wasn't necessary to come with me. Only with the persuasion of a close friend did I allow her to tag along—and was I grateful for her presence! Not that I couldn't bear the discomfort, but it did hurt and the actual test results were shattering. Having a hand to hold was so very important. Fortunately, I learned a lesson and made sure that my husband was by my side for the next two hysterosalpingograms I had in later years.*

Basic Survival Skills

If you are overwhelmed by what the infertility grind is, the question becomes: "How do I get through it?" It is helpful to remind yourself of other times in your life when you suffered a crisis and to remember how you worked through it. Everyone has a repertoire of coping skills developed over the years, and this is the time to pull out the ones that have served you well. I am sure you will have to learn some new ways to manage, but check out the resources you have already established. What in the past helped you to relieve anxiety when going through a difficult time? What were good escapes when circumstances became intolerable? What gave you a better understanding of your problem and how did you work through your feelings? The following coping skills may already be part of your repertoire, or perhaps they will be new ones you can cultivate.

Taking Control of Your Emotions

Whenever people experience crises in their lives, a sense of being out of control may prevail. Emotions take over and it is easy to feel as if you are on a runaway train, powerless to put on the brakes.

In the beginning, I really thought infertility was going to kill me. Depression would just take over my body and I would give in to it. It was as if someone was pounding me into the ground, and when I would try to get up, they would come back and give me one last blow.

It may seem impossible to you at first, but you *can* develop the skills to take control of these powerful feelings rather than allowing them to control you. Here are several ways to develop some mastery of those runaway emotions:

1. Recognize your feelings. Many people are clearly enraged by their situation but unable to admit to the intensity of their anger. If you do not realize what you are feeling or are overwhelmed by conflicting emotions, it is difficult to take control and do anything constructive with them. It also helps to know how people "normally" feel in handling infertility and to recognize that your responses are similar to those of others. Don't panic over the intensity of your feelings.

2. Learn to express the feelings in a direct and appropriate way. Storing up layer upon layer of anger, guilt, and frustration can have

serious emotional and physical repercussions. Counseling, to be discussed later, may be especially helpful in developing this skill.

3. Consider putting your thoughts and feelings into writing—keep a journal, send letters to friends, or write articles for a newsletter or magazine. It can not only provide a catharsis but also give a new perspective on your situation. Writing can be an outlet to work through the painful feelings that are keeping you stuck.

4. Develop the skill of using positive self-talk, or inner encouragement, when facing difficult situations. This can be used in combination with relaxation techniques to endure painful medical treatments, to handle the stress of learning critical test results, or to survive any anxiety-provoking situation that arises. For example, you might say, "Take a few deep breaths. I am upset, but I am in control and I can handle this."

5. Let yourself cry. There are going to be plenty of times when nothing else will help. You are allowed to fall apart now and then. It is healthy, normal, and can purge those miserable feelings.

6. Learn some relaxation techniques to deal with the everyday tension that is sure to arise. There are a number of popular books on the market today that deal specifically with handling stress (see the Bibliography). One such book, *The Relaxation Response* by Herbert Bensen, M.D., describes a relaxation technique derived from age-old practices in both Eastern and Western cultures. Some of his instructions are as follows:

1. Sit quietly in a comfortable position.

2. Close your eyes.

3. Deeply relax all your muscles, beginning at your feet and progressing up to your face. Keep them relaxed.

4. Breathe through your nose. Become aware of your breathing. As you breathe out, say the word "one" silently to yourself. For example, breathe in . . . out, "one"; in . . . out, "one"; etc. Breathe easily and naturally.

5. Continue for ten to twenty minutes. You may open your eyes to check the time, but do not use an alarm. When you finish, sit quietly for several minutes, at first with your eyes closed and later with your eyes opened. Do not stand up for a few minutes.

6. Do not worry about whether you are successful in achieving a deep level of relaxation. Maintain a passive attitude and permit relaxation to occur at its own pace. When distracting thoughts occur, try to ignore them by not dwelling upon them and return to repeating "one." With practice, the response should come with little effort. Practice the technique once or twice daily, but not within two hours after any meal, since the digestive processes seem to interfere with the elicitation of the Relaxation Response.[2]

Simple breathing exercises can actually be used anywhere in order to handle stress. I have done them in the car, at work, and in the bathroom at a party when I felt overwhelmed by anxiety. In a panic situation, or even under mild stress, your breathing rate tends to increase and your breath can become shallow. By focusing on your breathing and making a conscious effort to inhale and exhale in long, deep breaths through your nose or mouth, you can effectively relax. Allow your chest to expand fully and then slowly release the air, concentrating your thoughts only on the sensation of breathing. Several minutes of this can help immensely.

Another way of handling stress is through muscle relaxation exercises. One of these is a progressive relaxation technique that involves tensing and then relaxing all the body's major muscle groups, beginning with the face and head. An outline for progressive relaxation, described by Charlesworth and Nathan in their book *Stress Management*, is as follows:

I. Basic technique
   A. Separately tense your individual muscle groups.
   B. Hold the tension about five seconds.
   C. Release the tension slowly and at the same time silently say, "Relax and let go."
   D. Take a deep breath.
   E. As you breathe slowly out, silently say, "Relax and let go."
II. Muscle groups and exercises
   A. Head
      1. Wrinkle your forehead.
      2. Squint your eyes tightly.
      3. Open your mouth wide.
      4. Push your tongue against the roof of your mouth.

　　5. Clench your jaw tightly.
B. Neck
　　1. Push your head back into the pillow.
　　2. Bring your head forward to touch your chest.
　　3. Roll your head to your right shoulder.
　　4. Roll your head to your left shoulder.
C. Shoulders
　　1. Shrug your shoulders up as if to touch your ears.
　　2. Shrug your right shoulder up as if to touch your ear.
　　3. Shrug your left shoulder up as if to touch your ear.
D. Arms and hands
　　1. Hold your arms out and make a fist with each hand.
　　2. One side at a time: Push your hands down into the surface where you are practicing.
　　3. One side at a time: Make a fist, bend your arm at the elbow, tighten up your arm while holding the fist.
E. Chest and lungs
　　1. Take a deep breath.
　　2. Tighten your chest muscles.
F. Arch your back
G. Stomach
　　1. Tighten your stomach area.
　　2. Push your stomach area out.
　　3. Pull your stomach area in.
H. Hips, legs, and feet
　　1. Tighten your hips.
　　2. Push the heels of your feet into the surface where you are practicing.
　　3. Tighten your leg muscles below the knee.
　　4. Curl your toes under as if to touch the bottom of your feet.
　　5. Bring your toes up as if to touch your knees.[3]

The authors suggest that this technique be used twice each day for twenty minutes, if possible. Even brief practice sessions of five minutes or less, however, can be effective in reducing tension to a manageable level.

Another related technique described in *Stress Management* is the skill of body scanning in which you search your body rapidly for signs of tension areas. The procedure uses both steady breathing and instruction from the mind to "relax and let go" when you recognize particular areas under stress.[4] Chances are that certain parts of your body are prone to tension, such as your shoulders or stomach. Learning to identify your areas can help in quickly relaxing them.

Remember that learning to handle stress is a skill that will not happen overnight. It takes practice to become effective, so do not expect too much from yourself too quickly. If you want further assistance, stress management courses are given at local mental health centers, the YMCA, or adult education programs.

7. Recognize when situations cannot be changed no matter what you do. At times the best approach is to just sit back and take it as it comes. The sooner you accept the fact that infertility is stressful and that a certain amount of anxiety is part of the situation, the better off you will be. Trying to eliminate all the stress and control everything will only be counterproductive: it is impossible and it is likely to bring on even more frustration. Once you can say "I'm anxious and I've got a right to feel this way under the circumstances," it can lessen the pressure. One comment that most of my clients make when they enter counseling is that they feel incredibly nervous all the time, almost to the point of believing that they are "crazy." It is normal to feel "crazy" at times when you are struggling with infertility.

Combating Burnout: Redefining or Broadening Your Goals

In the midst of long-term infertility, people often use some or all of the following words to describe their state of mind and body: *exhausted, frustrated, overwhelmed, disinterested* (in anything but infertility), and *confused*. You could add to this list, I am sure. What all the words mean is that any joie de vivre you once felt has slipped away. You may feel that you and your life are a failure. Many go through the motions of everyday living, but that is all they are—just motions, with no enthusiasm behind them.

Pursuing infertility treatment can require so much energy and attention that it is easy to forget that life consists of more than producing a baby. You have probably heard the term *psychological burnout* applied to jobs or parenting. It may be defined as "a condition produced by working too hard for too long in a high-pressured situation," and is characterized by "physical and emotional exhaustion involving the development of negative self-concepts and negative attitudes towards work, life, and other people."[5] Those who develop burnout are often energetic perfectionists who struggle toward a single goal, often an exceptionally difficult one. It is possible that while struggling with infertility, you will suffer from burnout. Your goal is a difficult one, and there can seem, along the way, that only one type of success is possible—getting pregnant and delivering a healthy baby.

In order to combat the negative effects from burnout, you should both redefine and broaden your scope of goal setting. With regard to the infertility itself, establish tasks for yourself that are *manageable*. Break down the ultimate goal (whether pregnancy or adoption) into tasks that can be realistically accomplished in a short time. For example, instead of allowing yourself to be overwhelmed by the prospect of trying to adopt, decide that you will contact one attorney today or begin reading one book on adoption from the library. Don't try to do everything at once. Redefining your goals into manageable pieces can help with a sense of accomplishment.

In addition, begin to consider other goals (unrelated to infertility) to shoot for, whether on a short- or a long-term basis.

> *At one point in the infertility process when I was feeling particularly low, I made the decision that I had to do something to make me feel more competent, more worthwhile. I said to myself, "If you can't be a mother right now, then you might as well become the best damn teacher that you can." It was hard to get up the drive, but I eventually enrolled in a graduate program and started to work toward my master's degree. There's no question that my heart wasn't always in it, but in the end it made a critical difference in how I saw myself.*

If work- or education-related goals are too monumental to consider, there are other short-term aims worth pursuing. Redecorate that room you have wanted to change or start learning to play the piano. The worst that will happen is you may have to stop—and how bad would that be if you were pregnant? Creating the opportunity to feel a sense of accomplishment by attaining other goals in your life is well worth the effort. By broadening your investment in other goals, you may also, in the long run, be more emotionally capable of continuing the attack on infertility.

All of this means that you should make an effort to plan ahead. A major problem in experiencing infertility is the tendency to put everything in your life on hold—not planning vacations because you might become pregnant, not buying clothes because they won't fit if you get pregnant, not starting any new project because it might be interrupted by pregnancy, and so on.

> *I knew that we desperately needed to get away from all the pressures, but the thought of "missing a month" without treatment or seeing a doctor was intolerable. Sometimes I would sit for hours with a calendar in front of me trying to plot out future cycles to determine a "safe" time to go away.*

Handling any decision about the future becomes very difficult. Should you buy a house? Should you take that job promotion out of town? Is it a good idea to buy a two-seater car? This is a terrible way to live, but it is easy to fall into the trap. Many exist not in the present but totally in a fantasy future of pregnancy and parenthood.

> *Infertility has definitely put our lives on hold. Focusing on trying to get pregnant has isolated us, and I don't feel we're really living to fullest capacity. I think it is the uncertainty of not knowing whether pregnancy will occur that is the hardest to deal with. The day my doctor says we should give up will be a painful, but welcome, moment. We've lost control because we're "waiting" all the time—waiting for the next cycle, waiting to hear from the adoption agency, waiting to become parents.*

I am not sure that you can avoid altogether going through this aspect of infertility, but I do know that at some point you must stop. It is crucial to expand your vision and your goals, even if nothing compares with the importance of pregnancy. Look at your life and decide what you do have some control over and what can make a difference to you.

What Else Can Help?

When examining my own response to infertility and talking with hundreds of people going through the experience, it became clear to me that there are many ways of coping. The following ideas may help you find your own successful survival skills.

Leisure Activities—Have Some Fun!

It is hard to believe that life can be happy and rewarding when your greatest wish is unfulfilled. But remember: you had a life before all this started and other interests made you cheerful. Your leisure activities or special interests may not bring the degree of pleasure they offered in the past, but don't abandon any that you enjoy at all. They will not cure your infertility, but they are crucial to your self-esteem and your physical well-being.

Leisure activities can also be a terrific outlet for pent-up feelings, especially if they involve physical activity.

I've always been a runner and fortunately had the stamina to keep it up during my infertility treatment. It probably has been the primary factor in helping me keep my sanity. When everything looks totally bleak and I feel like crawling in a hole somewhere to die, I somehow find the energy to run or maybe it's to escape. Once out there, I can just "free associate," which is like being in my own private therapy session. It's a tremendous relief. Physically, too, it makes me feel healthy and alive at a time when all the infertility drugs are assaulting my body.

I cannot stress too much the importance of exercise in helping you cope. The benefits of an activity like running are both physical and psychological. The physical benefits are obvious, but you may be unaware of the psychological lift provided by aerobic exercise—any activity that uses oxygen to produce energy, such as jogging, swimming, racquetball, cycling, or jumping rope. First, it produces a sense of well-being—you feel better about yourself and your body, for it releases tension and relaxes the muscles. Exercise can clear your thoughts by giving you the opportunity to sort out the frustrations and problems that may be plaguing you. I have always found that I do my best thinking while running. I am more creative and better able to solve my problems. Sometimes exercisers, especially runners, develop an emotional high; it is not unusual to hear runners say, "I was cranky and in an intolerable mood before I left home to run, but I came back feeling at peace with myself and the world." Scientific evidence indicates that positive biochemical changes occur in the body as a result of aerobic exercise.

Another advantage of exercise is that it can provide a sense of independence and control over your life. You are not only doing something positive for yourself; you are achieving whatever goals you have set. This is a far cry from the frustration and failure of infertility. Leer, in an article "Running as an Adjunct to Psychotherapy," states that "for persons whose lives are beset by numerous 'loose ends,' engaging in regular exercise provides an opportunity to anticipate and successfully carry out a complete and constructive activity."[6] I know that running can be a powerful antidote to tension and depression and wholeheartedly recommend it.

On the other hand, there has been considerable publicity in recent years regarding the impact of long-distance running on the reproductive tract and fertility. For some women, it appears that running can decrease the amount of fatty tissue in the body below a normal level, thus leading to cessation of ovulation. Stangel, in *Fertility and Conception*, also suggests that the stress caused by long-distance running and even weight fluctuations that occur might contribute to temporary ovulation problems.[7] Be sure to discuss any extensive exercise plan with your doctor before proceeding.

Finding Something or Someone to Nurture

Many people find that having pets is a good emotional outlet for their desire to nurture and be needed. Even caring for plants can be rewarding. The idea of putting your energies and sensitivity into something alive, watching it respond and grow, can be satisfying amid all the frustration. Anyone who has had a pet knows how easily we attribute human characteristics to our animals.

My dog is like a little teddy bear to me. He is always there throughout the constant tears. I hug him, kiss him,

and dote on him. He is like another person to give me
support, only he doesn't talk back. I need his
unconditional love and he provides it.

Some infertile people have invested their time and emotions in foster care and found this to be a satisfying option while trying to start their own family. Doing this can also help you evaluate your infertility and approach resolution.

We will probably continue to try to have biological
children, but presently we are in the process of adopting
a little girl. What helped us make this decision was
having a child we were foster parents to and realizing
how much we could love someone else's biological
child.

If you investigate this possibility, however, you must be very careful to examine your feelings and motivations before making the commitment. How will you feel when you have to return a foster child to his birthparents? How would you handle the situation if you became pregnant while caring for a youngster? The child's best interests must be considered first, and it is important that you be honest with yourself in assessing the reasons for pursuing this option.

Laughter

As Barbara Eck Menning has said, "In the face of adversity, laughter is indeed the best medicine."[8] When you think objectively about all the craziness in struggling through infertility, you can acknowledge that some of the experiences really are funny. People who are able to maintain a sense of perspective and humor about it all have a wonderful advantage in surviving the infertility crisis. Although it is not a humorous subject, some of it is comic.

After several years of infertility treatment, enduring
practically every treatment in the book, my doctor
finally suggested a new drug approach that was just in
the research stage. It involved wearing a small infusion
pump around my waist which injected hormones

directly into my abdomen. When I actually thought
about the extent to which I'd gone to get pregnant, I
suddenly realized how absurd it was to be walking
around with this little gadget connected to me. I felt
like I'd become a "bionic" person hooked up to wires.
The whole experience became a joke, not because it was
an improper treatment, but because I could finally
laugh at myself and how ridiculous my life had
become. It was a relief to feel this way! I got through
two months of this therapy because I was able to stop
taking it so seriously.

Finding Support in Other Infertile People

Discovering other infertile individuals to talk to can make all the difference. Some of you may be comfortable enough to share your problem openly and develop your own contacts with others. But, more than likely, you have kept the problem to yourself, never recognizing that one of your colleagues or neighbors is experiencing the same thing. With 10 million infertile people in the United States, there are bound to be others around you who are suffering through a similar experience.

The most difficult feeling for me has been one of
aloneness. I had no idea there were so many people
dealing with infertility. I went to several doctors before
one even acknowledged the fact that we were not alone
in our sadness about not being able to have children.

One way of finding support is by joining a mutual help group in which people with a similar problem come together to share their experiences. One such group, founded in 1973, is RESOLVE, which describes itself as "a national, nonprofit charitable organization which offers counseling, referral, and support groups to people with problems of infertility, and education and assistance to associated professionals." Its educational component includes literature recommendations, speakers, fact sheets, and newsletters. Joining such an organization can provide a unique bonding experience because, for the first time, you may find understanding from others. No longer do you feel alone and different.

> *I found out, by joining RESOLVE, that everybody else cries as much as I do and that I am not losing my mind. I have also found out about procedures that need to be done and learned exactly what was going to happen to me. RESOLVE has been "someone to hold my hand," a reassurance that I am not alone.*

> *RESOLVE has been a life saver! It is an excellent information exchange and provides wonderful support groups. What a pleasure to be with a group of people who know your problem, instead of discussing diaper rash!*

Most who go through infertility do not want to be pitied, and yet sympathy from others in the fertile world often takes on an overtone of their feeling sorry for you. Finding support from an infertility group is far different because the others empathize, not just sympathize with your problems. They know what it is like when your best friend announces that she is pregnant. To laugh instead of cry with another person over the absurdities of early-morning temperature taking, or to share the pain of a miserable test result—that is what it is all about.

Many find that going to a group like RESOLVE provides a sense of relief if for no other reason than they learn that their feelings are shared by others. You do not have to explain yourself or constantly be on guard against hurtful comments. You can also begin to see your problems in a more realistic manner and learn to handle them more effectively.

Unfortunately, many have worries or misconceptions about joining a mutual help group that prevent them from making use of this valuable support. Some may feel they do not want to join because it will make them think more about their infertility problems and they would rather think less. But many who are infertile are obsessed about it, whether they participate in a group or not. The condition pervades your life, and trying to shut out the feelings will only make matters worse. The relief from joining a mutual help group can help *lessen* your tendency to dwell on infertility issues.

Some may feel that infertility is too personal or traumatic an experience to share with a group of people. My response is that it is too traumatic *not* to share with others. An organization like RESOLVE is not an encounter group or one that forces you to stand up and acknowledge "I am infertile." It is a safe, warm, supportive environment, neither aggressive nor confrontational.

Still others may not want to join a group because it gives them a feeling of futility. They may perceive such a group as being only for people who have hit the bottom and are without hope. That is far from the truth, for RESOLVE members are at all stages of infertility treatment, and many end up with successful pregnancies or adoptions because of information they obtained through the group.

But some will say that they are uncomfortable with groups—period. Although an organization like RESOLVE enjoys and needs the active participation of its members, a person can join, attend meetings, and benefit immensely without ever saying a word. The monthly programs are very informative, and if you are uneasy about attending meetings, the national and local newsletters can be very helpful. You can take from or offer to the group as much or as little as you want.

It is also important to note that RESOLVE is for both women and men. As one man said:

> RESOLVE *was helpful to me, although not to my wife. I found a lot of benefit by reading the* RESOLVE *newsletters and sharing experiences with others at the meetings. Several years ago, early in our infertility, I remember talking to someone at a Serono symposium about how infertility can adversely affect a relationship. At the time, my wife and I scoffed at the idea—we were better, we could endure. We had already been trying two years and hadn't gotten divorced. Little did we know then that we were just getting started in the ordeal. We have since divorced, but I have continued my membership with* RESOLVE. *I have learned very much about infertility from* RESOLVE *and what it did to my marriage.*

It is very easy to believe that nothing except a successful pregnancy will make any difference in enduring your infertility. That, however, is not necessarily true. A group can make a difference for many people, and a few meetings would seem worth a try. If you only want a few questions answered, both national RESOLVE and local chapters offer a telephone counseling service. Feel free to call with any concerns regarding tests, treatment, referrals, medications, the groups, or any other aspect of infertility. Remember that building walls around you may seal off some pain, but it also effectively seals off the opportunity for understanding, guidance, and support.

The Role of Professional Counseling

People decide that professional counseling might be beneficial for many reasons. Some feel that infertility has taken too great a toll on themselves or on their relationships with others, and they feel powerless to turn the situation around on their own. Others have few supports and need someone to turn to who can provide guidance and support. Still others find that they need the objective help of a third person in handling the many decisions of infertility. A common belief is that only mentally unstable people get involved with counseling, but that is not true. To the contrary, those who seek professional help display strength and motivation in wanting to improve their lives.

Counseling provides an opportunity for individuals and couples to express safely and work through the multitude of feelings that can overwhelm them in infertility. It does not necessarily delve into your past or dredge up painful secrets. Nor is the counselor out to prove that you are psychologically causing your own infertility.

In the beginning, counseling can provide a greater understanding of the medical problems involved and set a time frame for further investigation and treatment. It can also be immensely beneficial in relieving stress. Although research has not shown that stress causes infertility, it is clear that the body does not function optimally under conditions of severe anxiety. The relief of stress through counseling, then, may be a useful adjunct to medical treatment. Counseling can also aid in the resolution process by clarifying needs and desires and assessing the available alternatives. If it becomes evident that a couple will not be able to have biological children, counseling can help them deal with that significant loss.

Couples may find counseling particularly helpful when the problems of infertility have affected their marital relationship. With the security and guidance of an objective third person, they can talk more openly about their feelings, understand each other better, and recognize how infertility has affected their relationship. A professional counselor can point out destructive patterns of behavior and communication and help develop alternative ways of relating. Often, couples learn to view their relationship and their predicament from a different perspective.

> *My husband and I have been in counseling for eight months. I feel that if we didn't go, I'd be in a padded cell somewhere. Our counselor has been great, answering questions that our doctor has no time for, as well as working with the doctor on our case.*

> *I finally went for counseling and found that it helped me deal with my anger, raise my self-esteem, and come to grips with my life. It brought me understanding and acceptance.*

> *My husband and I have been to two counseling sessions in preparation for AID. It was valuable for me in that the counselor said enough to push me over an edge that I needed to move over. It helped me confront my emotions in the light of day. It also was the beginning of my openness about infertility. As a couple, it helped both of us understand and accept the differences in our reactions to infertility.*

It may be frightening to even consider the idea of counseling, let alone call for an appointment.

> *I have considered going for counseling, but I think my husband rejects the idea. I think I just have to make the first move. I suppose going would be admitting that I (we) have a problem, a large problem. I like to think that I am able to work through my problems alone, not have to share them with other people, though other times I feel that is just what I need. I guess I will get around to it eventually, the longer this "problem" exists.*

Such reservations are not uncommon. People also fear how much they will need to share and how they may be perceived by the counselor or others who know of their problems. As anxiety provoking as it may be initally, the experiences quoted earlier attest to how helpful counseling can be.

Two important points should be mentioned in discussing the value of counseling. First, it is essential that the professional you select is knowledgeable about infertility and has worked with infertile individuals and couples. I know several people who have had negative experiences with professionals who were not familiar with infertility. Contact your physician or RESOLVE to get an appropriate referral. The second point is that, unfortunately, many people wait until they or their relationship have hit rock bottom before considering counseling. It can be far more successful if used earlier in treatment, rather than facing it as a last-ditch effort when a marriage has already fallen apart.

Hope—Friend or Enemy?

Hope is a funny thing. When you feel that you are absolutely at the end of your rope, it can suddenly appear, bringing with it a seemingly magical sense of cheer. It will permit your imagination to soar, unbounded by painful realities. The problem is, however, that hope is also fragile—swelling one moment and shattered the next.

I always found it perplexing to figure out just how much hope was realistic, and I would ask myself, "Am I only fooling myself? Am I living in a dream world?" There are times when you allow hope to surge within you, imbuing you with a sense of optimism and confidence. On other occasions, you approach it more cautiously, fearful of its destructive side. Certainly, allowing hope to flourish also means you are vulnerable, for the stage is set for possible disappointment.

> *There have been times when I've looked at hope as my enemy, some kind of cruel monster. My hopes would be raised only to be squelched with a terrible test result or the arrival of my period. At times, I swore I'd never dream again. They say "the higher you fly, the harder you fall." It's probably true. But, on the other hand, I'm not sure I could survive without that ability to hope. And, in the end, I guess the failures will always hurt anyway, with or without hope.*

Hope becomes dangerous or destructive only when it fails to acknowledge reality. Infertility patients and their doctors alike need eventually to admit when hope is unrealistic and has become a denial of an impossible situation.

Taking a Vacation from Treatment

As I write this, I realize that I am speaking from hindsight; I probably wouldn't have taken the advice I am about to offer when I was struggling with my own infertility. For taking a vacation from treatment sounds terrific in theory but may be extremely hard to accomplish. I was never able to try it, but I hope that some of you will recognize the value and be able to make use of it.

Taking a rest from treatment, whether for a month or a year, can be liberating to those who have come to a breaking point. Not to have to endure the tension and depression of regular treatment provides such a relief that many are happily shocked by the feeling. It offers a time, free of infertility obsession, to once again get in touch with yourself—who you are, what you enjoy, and the variety of things you want out of life. And how easy it is to forget that there is a life out there that has nothing to do with children or getting pregnant. A vacation from treatment can provide a new, more positive, perspective on life just by giving you the opportunity to do something other than take temperatures and run to doctor appointments. And you are reminded that there is a part of you that is successful and fun to be with.

> *During our infertility, we took several exciting trips to wonderful, faraway places. It was wonderful to escape the rigors of treatment for a short while and the planning was an exhilarating outlet for me, probably the only time I wasn't dwelling on my problems. The trips brought out my sense of wanderlust—a special part of me that often got lost in the grind of daily life and a part of me that I really liked.*

Taking a vacation from treatment will give you a chance to reassess your goals and take a clear look at what you have been putting yourself through month after month. It is difficult to have a rational perspective when you are running from one doctor's appointment to the next. If nothing else, the time will raise your spirits and energize you enough to get back into the rat race again.

I chose not to take a break because I was afraid of "losing a month." Not until later did I realize my deeper fear that if I stopped I might never have the stamina to begin again. As one woman said:

> *When we made the decision to adopt, it was not, at the time, a real end-all resolution for me. I was looking forward to it and was comfortable with the choice but, in the depths of my mind, I assumed that I would soon return to infertility treatment, forever pursuing the goal of actually having a child. I even remember telling my doctor, at the time of the adoption, that I'd be back in a few months. Well, it's been almost three years now and I have no intention of ever returning to that struggle. I don't think I could ever immerse myself again in that mental anguish. What started as a rest in my treatment became a total resolution and a lifetime decision. What a sense of peace!*

Remember that, at some point, you must recognize what you are doing to yourself in this stressful situation.

Yes-infertility has devastated your life.

Yes-it is unfair.

Yes-it is a situation that is largely out of your control.

That is the uncomfortable reality and it is very hard to face. But keep in mind that you cannot be a failure at something over which you have no control. Infertility will not destroy your entire life unless you allow it to. Infertility can bring out the worst in people, but it can also generate the best—if you let it.

Infertility and Religion

The Role of Religion

For thousands of years, people have turned to religion to explain and ascribe meaning to circumstances beyond their control. They have derived a sense of security and hope from the belief that the mysteries of the universe, although beyond human understanding, are within the control of some all-encompassing power.

Religion has furnished answers to the perplexing questions of the significance of human beings in the universe and why events happen as they do. It has comforted people in times of tragedy and offered principles by which to live, providing a system of values and a sense of direction, especially during times of crisis. People have found in religion a sense of community. The church has been a place to belong, where they could share their thoughts and feelings not only with God but with others of similar faith.

It is not surprising then that religion can be of value to people experiencing infertility. They need a sense of hope, and their faith may supply this. It can also offer security and provide meaning—both so desperately needed during this crisis. Many speak, too, of how comforting it is to feel loved by God when they are feeling so wretched about themselves.

> *I may not understand justice in this world but, through my religious faith, there is hope of justice and peace in life after death. I feel that God has a special purpose for me, so special that I will be more than just a common housewife and mother. Soon He will show me what my special purpose is.*

Sometimes, however, people expect from religion what may be impossible—that all their prayers will be granted. When this does not happen, they must grapple with anger and disappointment. For them religion may become a mixed blessing, as its positive values are mingled with feelings of disillusionment. There is often confusion and pain as these people try to reconstruct their beliefs and maintain their faith.

> *My religion has been both a blessing and a torment. A blessing because I have someone to talk to and am able to pray for babies—that gives me some hope. A torment because I'm supposed to trust and accept the will of God; yet I'm disappointed and discouraged month after month. I think if I had been a better person, God would not be punishing me. And yet I know in my heart that He doesn't "punish" people and that He is a forgiving God. I'm constantly being tested in my faith. Sometimes I become so angry with God that I feel guilty. Yet I can't imagine going through all this without my religious faith.*

Searching for Meaning

Why Me?

> *Five years have passed since the glad and hopeful time when we began to try to become pregnant. Our expectations ran high; we were ready to become parents. Months passed, a year, our prayers unanswered. I felt, surely, God must hear. As time went on my doubts grew. I felt forsaken, barren, cursed. God seemed to me like a stern, frowning judge. Infertility felt like a cruel sentence, yet somehow deserved.[1]*

Many people grow up with a sense of righteousness and fairness—that if they are good, moral individuals, they will be rewarded for their endeavors. The Bible is filled with passages that encourage this belief, and many desperately try to maintain its truth.

Most people would also like to believe that there is order in the world and that life makes sense. But this vision usually collapses after an experience with tragedy.

> *My religious beliefs have suffered as a result of my*
> *infertility and other events over which I had no control.*
> *In the last year and a half, my father-in-law died, my*
> *mother died, and I found out that I have only a 50*
> *percent chance of ever having a child. I can't help*
> *looking at God and wondering how He could let all*
> *this happen to me—what did I do to deserve this? As a*
> *result, my prayers have become rather empty. I am*
> *trying to regain my faith and renew my trust in God,*
> *but it's hard.*

Anyone who has lost a loved one or watched another endure a crushing blow can relate to the agonizing question of how fair the world is. Even before experiencing infertility, you probably knew of people—good, kind people—struck down by tragedy.

> *As an adolescent, I would frequently become embroiled*
> *in religious arguments over the meaning of suffering*
> *and how such suffering relates to a person's morality*
> *and religious convictions. At that time, it was an*
> *intellectual exercise and good for some heated debates.*
> *But, when infertility hit me, it suddenly became a very*
> *real and excruciatingly painful issue. Why was I*
> *suffering?*

Kushner asked in his best-selling book, "Why do bad things happen to good people?" What is fair about a seventeen-year-old having an abortion or a twenty-five-year old conceiving her sixth unplanned child whom she cannot afford to feed and clothe, and all the while, you are struggling to have a family and encountering roadblocks every inch of the way? It is impossible not to question, "Why me?"

Trying to reconcile your infertility with a belief in the existence of God may be extremely difficult, especially if you believe that God is the creator of all life events, good or bad. Judith Stigger has written a book entitled *Coping with Infertility*, which deals with infertility from a theological point of view. She lists four theories of suffering that she has found to be commonly believed by infertile Christians:

1. Infertility as "punishment for sin"
2. Infertility as a means to prepare individuals "for the rigors of service as [God's] ambassadors to others"
3. Infertility "as a message from God to rethink one's life plans"
4. Infertility as a form of suffering that is "not a direct message from God," but rather an act of God that is "beyond human understanding"[2]

Those who view God as a stern, judgmental authority who dictates the final destination of heaven or hell will most likely see infertility as a deserved punishment, since everyone has "sinned" at some point in his or her life. Others who need to feel that God is a power that supervises and controls the world will presumably feel that everything that occurs in life has a purpose ordained by God. Therefore, suffering through infertility, for these people, must carry with it some meaning—perhaps to teach a lesson or to make you see life from a different perspective or to turn you into a better person.

Finally, those who cannot find any meaning in their infertility but believe that God is all-knowing and omnipotent may decide that their infertility is part of a larger plan they do not have the capacity to understand. For many, these beliefs do offer comfort.

> *I always had faith that my belief in God would help me through anything. I always thought that if you prayed hard enough for something, you would get it. But when you wholeheartedly go to church everyday and then find out that your tubes are blocked after just having a tuboplasty, it is real easy to become an atheist. I have recently begun to look at things differently and have come to a lot of new conclusions. I realize now that God has a reason for all of this. And if being a parent is part of this plan, that's great! But, if his plan for me is that I am to be childless, I must accept that, too. Now when I pray, I pray that I'll accept what is ahead, I pray for strength to cope, and I pray*

for direction. I'm letting God take control of my life.
I'm putting it in His hands because He knows what is
best for me.

All these views trouble me because they presume that God is in total control of people's lives, ushering in pain or joy as He sees fit. As Kushner says,

> *The idea that God gives people what they deserve, that*
> *our misdeeds cause our misfortune, is a neat and*
> *attractive solution to the problem of evil at several*
> *levels, but it has a number of severe limitations. As we*
> *have seen, it teaches people to blame themselves. It*
> *creates guilt even where there is no basis for guilt. It*
> *makes people hate God, even as it makes them hate*
> *themselves. And most disturbing of all, it does not even*
> *fit the facts.*[3]

I feel that the individual's perception of God relates to one's vision of self and one's capacity as a human being. Those who find religion to have a positive effect in their lives during infertility look upon God as a source of strength, solace, and growth, not as a power that punishes or rewards. A low sperm count, then, is not a decree from God that they have sinned but a medical problem that requires strength to handle.

Thus, there is no answer to the question "Why me?" despite the efforts to find one. As I gradually accepted infertility for what it is (a medical condition preventing a person from having children) and renewed my self-esteem (I was a good person, despite my faults, and I would make a good mother), I recognized that it is not a question of blame and that infertility has no "meaning." It is part of life—and life is not always fair.

It is not the *reason* infertility has affected you that brings meaning and purpose; it is the *consequence* of infertility—what you decide to make of it. If you decide that the problem is going to destroy you, your marriage, and your relationships with others, then that, sadly, is what will happen. But if you decide to pick up the pieces and move on, with greater appreciation of yourself, your spouse, and your loved ones, then the tragedy will have some redeeming value.

Religious Crisis and Disillusionment

Your religious beliefs may pass through several stages as your attitudes toward yourself and your predicament change. Those who believe in God commonly question not only His intentions but also His existence. Some end up finding stronger bonds with their religion, but others are unable to reconcile their pain with their beliefs.

> *I began to wonder if there really was a God. Then I felt that He must be postponing me for some reason. Was I really worthy of a child? When I finally did become pregnant, I began to bleed and all I could do was bargain ("If you let me hold my baby, I'll . . ."). Throughout all this, my beliefs have changed and I've gained more faith. But I still don't understand why some people are infertile.*

> *I was Catholic when I first became aware of my infertility. Now I don't know what I am, except confused. At first, I felt a lot of guilt (Catholicism likes it that way). I thought I must have done something terrible that God wouldn't let us be parents. I prayed all the time. I did novenas. I called prayer lines, and still the results were the same—nothing. One morning I woke up after praying so hard the night before that it wore me out, and got rid of anything religious in my sight—rosary beads, pictures, novena cards. Since then, I have not prayed once. I think God is a name people use to blame things on, good or bad. I have absolutely no proof that there is a God and, until I do, I don't believe in one. My mother is extremely religious and she's been driving me batty. She says if God wants you to have kids then He will provide you with them. I don't swallow that one anymore. I would definitely say my beliefs have changed.*

Infertile individuals who feel guilty because of their inability to conceive are very likely to experience a phase in which they try to atone for transgressions and strike bargains with God. But when all the prayers, penance, and "good behavior" fail, their rage is likely to intensify. Some may complain bitterly that God is unjust or that religion is a sham. At this point, it is not unusual for an infertile person to feel that nothing in life is worth striving for and all faith may be lost.

> *I was raised (as my husband was) a Roman Catholic. My family prays for me, gives me prayer cards and prayer books, and tells me to go to church. But every month my period comes again, and such and such a saint has let me down. With that kind of attitude, I suppose I don't have much faith. I already feel that my body has let me down and I can deal with that tangible aspect, but religion has not been a help. When I am very down I can pray, but I feel hypocritical.*

Also common during infertility is the wish for a miracle. Many infertile people find themselves, in desperation, praying for one, regardless of their faith. Then when the miracle does not occur, the person can be overcome by depression or cynicism: "How could God create all those wonderful miracles when all I want is a child like everyone else?"

Many people with whom I have spoken had to pass through this stage of doubt and disillusionment before ultimately finding strength from their religious faith. Often, this has meant their redefining the meaning of God rather than disclaiming any value in religion.

> *In the beginning, religion was a big help since I felt that if I prayed enough I would certainly get pregnant. When that didn't happen, my beliefs grew weaker and I was very angry with God. How could He let this happen? Despite these feelings, I continued to feel better when I prayed. What I've since learned is that I need to pray to have God help me cope, rather than to make me pregnant. My beliefs have changed in that I now feel that maybe God doesn't control every aspect of our lives, and that events like infertility are accidents of nature rather than God's direct doing.*

Finding Strength

> *My religious beliefs have grown stronger because of my*
> *experience with infertility. I could not have survived*
> *had it not been for my belief in God and the support*
> *both He and my husband have given me. I do question*
> *things more, asking "Why me?" many times a month,*
> *but I try to think positively. I pray daily for strength*
> *and to know God's will regarding having or not having*
> *children.*

Finding strength is at the core of the infertility experience—strength to confront, to persevere, and eventually to overcome and accept. It is important that you strive for this strength—whether through your religious faith, the loving support of family and friends, or your inner determination—to meet the many challenges of the infertility process. I believe that God's power is reflected in people's loving relationships with others and their capacity to face challenge and grow. God, as a symbol of strength, love, and creativity, lies within everyone, and that is the power you can summon when hit with tragedy.

For some people, a personal faith in God serves as a tremendous support throughout infertility, especially when that faith implies an unconditional love from God.

> *I have recently begun attending church more regularly*
> *and feel better about myself, now understanding that*
> *God did not punish me or my wife. It's good to know*
> *that God loves you whether you are fertile or not, or*
> *whether you are a parent or not. I am just sorry I was*
> *not more actively engaged in religious support at the*
> *time we were going through our most trying years.*
> *Everything then focused on medical concerns—not*
> *emotional or social. That was a mistake.*

As Stigger notes in *Coping with Infertility*, "Faith does not offer an exemption from the onslaught of painful emotions, but it does provide a framework within which to process those emotions."[4] For many infertile people, religion provides the opportunity to express their painful feelings to God—they can talk to God if others don't seem to care or understand. Religion also offers the chance to confess "sins" that may be the source of guilt and then to be forgiven by a loving God. Many find this "cleansing" to be of great benefit in learning to accept their infertility.

For some, the camaraderie of their religious group provides their strongest feeling of support.

> *Our religion is Unitarian-Universalist, a liberal*
> *Christian denomination, which fortunately allows for a*
> *wide divergence among its members. Most of our*
> *friends are associated with our U.U. fellowship. They are*
> *very helpful; thus, religion is helpful.*

For others, religious study increases their faith and brings them closer to their spouse.

> *[My husband] and I had been doing individual Bible*
> *study, but we learned the importance of incorporating*
> *family Bible study into our married routine. God has*
> *drawn us closer as we read and discuss His Word*
> *together. It has been a good opportunity to talk about*
> *our infertility and God's plan for us.*[5]

Prayer can be valuable, not because God will necessarily hear and change your life, but because it can help you express and work through painful emotions, restoring your self-esteem and your belief that you can weather difficult times. As Kushner says,

> *We can't pray that He make our lives free of problems;*
> *this won't happen, and it is probably just as well. We*
> *can't ask Him to make us and those we love immune*
> *to disease, because He can't do that. We can't ask him*
> *to weave a magic spell around us so that bad things*
> *only happen to other people, and never to us. People*
> *who pray for miracles usually don't get miracles, any*
> *more than children who pray for bicycles, good grades,*
> *or boyfriends get them as a result of praying. But*
> *people who pray for courage, for strength to bear the*

unbearable, for the grace to remember what they have
left instead of what they have lost, very often find their
prayers answered. They discover that they have more
strength, more courage than they ever knew themselves
to have. Where did they get it? I would like to think
that their prayers helped them find that strength. Their
prayers helped them tap hidden reserves of faith and
courage which were not available to them before.[6]

I know that I have grown through my infertility struggle—not
because that was the purpose of my suffering but because of what I
made of the experience. I will never know "why" my husband and I
are infertile, but the reason no longer matters. Through faith, determination, and the love of others, I have moved beyond that to
recognize and appreciate the positives that have resulted from the
pain. The final truth is that infertility, like any crisis in your life, can
promote growth as well as destroy it. It is what you make of the
experience that determines the outcome.

How Various Religions View Infertility

One of my earliest memories of childhood was going to
church. It seemed like we were always going to church.
There, parents would bring their children and learn
more about God. Little did I realize that many things I
had learned as a child would cause me so many
problems in my adult life.

It is not unusual for couples to retreat from their religion when
experiencing infertility because of the pressures they feel are im-
posed by the doctrine and the messengers of their faith. Although
there are wide variations in beliefs and acceptable conduct even
within a given faith, some ideas common to various religions will be
discussed here.

Often religions teach that a woman's only role and significance
lies in her ability to create new life.

One of the things that caused me so much pain was
that, as a woman in a fundamentalist Christian

community, I was taught I had no rights, just one basic
purpose—wife and mother. When I began to realize that
I fell short of this expectation, I knew I had to find an
answer to my questions. Was I really a woman? Why
was I even born if I could not fulfill my basic
responsibility? Why was God punishing me?

In early religious writings, an infertile woman was called "barren," a word with associations of arid, unproductive land. She was therefore of limited value. A woman unable to bear children might easily take on these same feelings today, believing that her only purpose in life is in vain. She might even, by extension, think of herself as a "non-person," especially if she has no strong sense of self in other areas of her life. Some religions explicitly state that a woman's infertility is grounds for annulment of a marriage (although, interestingly the same does not apply to a man's infertility).

Many religious teachings make a direct correlation between a woman's worthiness and her ability to bear children; that is, conception is granted only to those who are deserving. In the Bible, for example, many women unable to bear children ultimately conceive only because they are found worthy in God's eyes. With such messages, it is no wonder that guilt can arise so easily in those who are infertile.

In Orthodox Judaism, marriage and family cannot be separated, for without the existence of children, a union between two people is unfulfilled. The Old Testament states that a couple must "be fruitful and multiply" (Genesis 1:28), a commandment that allows little, if any, room for choice. Infertility of a person within the Orthodox community is conspicuous since it is expected by all that procreation will follow soon after marriage. Pressures may be even greater on the infertile Orthodox couple because their community tends to be a fixed, closed group that may not allow them to withdraw or to alter their social contacts. The belief in producing large families means that the infertile person is likely to be surrounded by many youngsters and have to endure lengthy discussions on raising children.

Making matters even more difficult for the infertile Orthodox couple are the many rules among the most religious that apply to the couple's sexual relationship. Intercourse is forbidden during the woman's menstrual period as well as for the next seven days. This is part of the law of family purity, which is still a basic tenet in the Orthodox Jewish faith. After this period, the woman immerses herself in a mikvah, or special ritual bath; then intercourse is permissible again. These rules of niddah (the time when a woman is sexually unavailable) may interfere with the time of ovulation and thus can prevent conception from occurring.[7]

When medical treatment is being sought or if there is a need to alter these rules, the Orthodox Jewish couple must first obtain permission from a rabbi. Permission is frequently granted, but if it is not, the couple faces a major problem, for the rabbi's decision is final.[8] Some couples choose not to seek rabbinical permission because of embarrassment or fear of rejection, but in that case they must deal with the guilt that often ensues. Many rabbis, however, are open and knowledgeable about the subject of infertility, and they may be helpful to couples facing the problem.

The Mormon religion, too, can create pressure for the infertile couple because of its strong emphasis on family.

No other success can compensate for failure in the home.

Families are forever.

Our children are our jewels in the crown of eternal life.[9]

These quotations all reflect the Mormon church's structure of belief, and perhaps exemplify feelings shared by many of you, regardless of your religion. It is difficult to be part of a close, sharing community when you are unable to participate in such an integral aspect of its life and faith.

> *I can no longer go to church because I get too depressed. Everything seems to be centered around family life and I find I get emotional just seeing a baby with a young couple.*

Establishing a family is so important to Mormons that women, in their early years, receive elaborate instruction on motherhood. What pressure to be trained to be a good mother, only to be denied the opportunity by infertility. The Mormon church is supportive of adoption, but it is handled within the confines of the faith, and often entails long waiting lists and stringent requirements.

Fewer treatment choices are available to infertile couples who follow closely the doctrines of their religion. For example, artificial insemination with use of a donor's sperm is not approved by the Roman Catholic church and, therefore, would not be an option for a strict observer of that faith. It is perceived to be a form of adultery and any offspring of conception through AID would be branded illegitimate. The Lutheran church shares this view, although the majority of other Protestant faiths consider the technique acceptable. Within Orthodox Judaism, not only is donor insemination frowned upon, but the use of masturbation in other procedures is also condemned.[10]

Despite sanctions against such techniques, some clergymen in these faiths have given approval for use in certain situations. For example, among Orthodox Jews, masturbation might be approved if sperm cannot be obtained in any other manner and if all the sperm are utilized.

The newer techniques of in vitro fertilization, surrogate parenting, and embryo transfer present even greater religious dilemmas because, to many, they represent the "manipulation" of human life. Both the Roman Catholic and the Orthodox Jewish religions have opposed these medical advances, whereas the Protestant and Reformed Jewish faiths have been more supportive of their use. Surrogate parenting has brought about the strongest opposition, not only because it involves a third party (and thus is perceived as intruding upon the sanctity of marriage), but because some consider it a form of "baby-selling."

Often, these constraints set off a crisis: the person reaches out to religion and medicine, but they are in conflict, and the person is faced with a painful choice. To solve this dilemma, some struggle to separate their religious faith from the doctrines of their church.

> As a practicing Catholic, my church didn't seem to support me, but I think my religious faith did. Birth control is forbidden, yet if I ever conceived again, the baby would most likely die (due to genetic factors, as did our first child). AID is also not approved of by the church, although a priest we consulted on this point seemed to indicate that this was a matter of individual conscience. While I have learned to be comfortable about using birth control since our baby's death, I was never totally comfortable about attempting AID. I know

that the church's stand has had something to do with
my feelings. On the other hand, with regard to religious
faith, I do believe that my daughter who died is with
God and that comforts me. Ironically, our son was
adopted through a Catholic agency.

Many people seem to be able to maintain their religious faith and to derive strength from their relationship with God without feeling they must follow every rule laid down by their church. Their consciences allow them to do what is right and comfortable for them, not necessarily what is dictated by the church.

From a practical standpoint, it is important that you find a physician who understands your religious background and will adhere to the beliefs and guidelines you present. The internal struggle between the demands of religion and medicine can be difficult enough without the additional pressure of an unaware or insensitive physician. Make sure that you present any religious constraints early in the relationship with your doctor so that these concerns can be openly discussed.

The Doctor-Patient Relationship

*A free-flowing communication between doctor and
patient implies a humanistic, caring physician and a
confident, assertive patient. The problem is to get each
of them from where they are to where they ought to be.*[1]

Choosing a Physician

The relationship with your physician during infertility is exceedingly
important and probably different from your encounters with doctors
in the past. The main difference is that infertility rarely involves just
a few appointments. It can become a long-lasting relationship in
which you invest much time and emotion. The physician frequently
becomes a person to whom you attribute superhuman qualities and
imagine to be a potential savior. Sensitive information, of which no
one else is aware, is often shared, and you are likely to display gut-
level emotions that few others may know exist. Certainly, it is not a
"usual" doctor-patient relationship.

Serious decision making, you will find, becomes a constant part
of the infertility experience, starting with the selection of a doctor.
Knowledge about infertility is increasing all the time, so it is important that the physician you consult is keeping abreast of the new
information. This means you should seek a doctor who was trained
in and now specializes in infertility. The choice of a doctor is complicated by the fact that infertility touches on a number of medical
specialties—infertility specialists may be found in the fields of gynecology, urology, or endocrinology. Each may be knowledgeable about
only a specific aspect of reproduction, so that eventually you may
need to consult more than one physician. What is best is to find a

group of professionals who work together as an infertility team or a doctor who can coordinate treatment, making the appropriate referrals.

It is not unusual, among a group of infertility patients, to hear numerous accounts of patient mismanagement, from both a physical and an emotional point of view. Here are two examples:

The first doctor I went to was a cold, uncompassionate person who refused to give me the time of day. After he operated on me (for six hours), he disappeared from the hospital for five days without even leaving someone to tell me and my husband what he had found. During regular office appointments, he often refused to answer my questions and what little discussion we had could only be accomplished while my feet were in the stirrups. His final words to me during the last appointment I ever had with him were "What do you expect? You have so many medical problems anyway—how do you think you'll ever get pregnant!" I was more than devastated.

I've had eight doctors in a two-year time period and only three of them were the doctors I needed. By this I mean that Doctors 1 and 2 informed me that they couldn't find anything wrong with me and suggested that I relax. Doctor 3 diagnosed me within an hour and began treatment which led to a pregnancy that aborted spontaneously at eight weeks. By that time, Doctor 3 had accepted a more prestigious position at a local teaching hospital and had to dump his caseload. Doctor 4 was insensitive to the physical pain I had and, instead, put me on painkillers. Doctor 5 told me a pregnancy was hopeless. Doctor 6 understood that I was in acute chronic pain because there was something terribly wrong with my pelvic organs. He referred me to Doctor 7 for a surgical consultation. Doctor 7 told me to lose twenty pounds, go back on Clomid, and pursue adoption. He also asked if I was certain my previous pregnancy was caused by my husband. Doctor 8 finally diagnosed a large ovarian cyst, pelvic adhesions caused

> *by an acute chlamydia infection, scarred tubes, and a*
> *retroflexed uterus. Doctors 3, 6, and 8 were very*
> *sensitive and understanding. The others seemed to resent*
> *the fact that I was assertive and that I had the right to*
> *participate in my treatment. Of those, two doctors*
> *refused to let me see my own records and were very*
> *nasty about giving my records to a new doctor.*

Experiences like these are well worth trying to avoid! But to do so requires serious investigation. Finding a competent physician in the field of infertility may not be an easy task, especially if you do not live near a large metropolitan area.

Most people who suspect an infertility problem will initially contact their family physician or gynecologist. He or she is likely to make such basic recommendations as keeping a temperature chart and having a semen analysis made in order to detect any obvious fertility problem. If these procedures do not shed light on the problem or if pregnancy still does not occur within the next three to six months, it would be beneficial to find an infertility specialist. You can ask your physician for a recommendation or contact the following referral sources:

1. Both national and local RESOLVE chapters. The national office can be contacted at RESOLVE, Inc., P.O. Box 474, Belmont, MA 02178; telephone (617) 484-2424. There are also forty local chapters throughout the United States. If there is a local group near you, it may be helpful to attend a meeting and speak with members about their experiences with various doctors.

2. The American Fertility Society, 1608 13th Avenue, Suite 101, Birmingham, AL 35256; telephone (205) 933-7222.

3. The American Medical Society. Contact local chapters listed in your telephone directory.

4. Others with whom you are acquainted who have a history of infertility. These persons can be an excellent source of information regarding a doctor's expertise in handling the patient, including accessibility, sensitivity, and communication skills.

5. The telephone directory. By checking the Yellow Pages, you can gather the names of physicians who advertise their interest in infertility. They may be listed under their medical specialty of gynecology, urology, or endocrinology. This will not tell you anything about their medical expertise, but it will give you a starting point for further investigation.

Once you have obtained names of several physicians and are trying to make your selection, consider the following points (a brief telephone call may answer some of your questions):

1. Do not hesitate to question a physician's background and training: Where did the doctor train and did this include specific training in infertility? How long has he or she been specializing in infertility? You can also ask how much of his or her practice is geared to infertility, the number of patients being treated, and success rates. Don't be afraid to ask—you are the consumer.

2. Inquire about fees. Infertility treatment can be very expensive, and you don't need the shock of an exhorbitant bill. Check your medical insurance to determine what kind of procedures are covered. If money is a problem for you, speak to the doctor about the possibility of making special arrangements. Many physicians are sensitive to this difficulty and willing to help.

3. Take into consideration a physician's location. Frequent appointments are often necessary, so you need to know how easily you can make trips, especially if they are to be fitted into a work schedule. Also inquire about the days and times that appointments are available.

4. Ask others about a physician's personality and bedside manner. Although you need to find a doctor with significant medical expertise, you also want someone with emotional sensitivity. Some physicians are frankly "cold fish" who do not have the ability to establish rapport with their patients. Others may be burned out by the frustrations of the field and the emotional demands of their patients. Remember, too, that not all doctors are going to relate well to all patients. The question of personality is

certainly an important issue, meaning you need to find an individual with whom *you* feel comfortable.

5. Assess a physician's knowledge of and comfort with the emotional elements of infertility. This can best be done by speaking with others who have consulted this doctor and by checking to see if he or she is aware of RESOLVE and supportive of it. Infertility cannot be effectively treated without an awareness of and sensitivity to its emotional aspects.

Unfortunately, some physicians are unaware of or uncomfortable with the emotional factors and, therefore, do not take them into consideration in treating their patients. They may cavalierly dismiss any emotional difficulties as being unimportant or they may imply that a patient's agitation is interfering with the medical treatment. One woman I know tried on several occasions to tell her doctor how depressed she had been, but he routinely answered, "Don't worry—you'll get pregnant." This does not mean that all physicians must be "Dr. Welbys" and must themselves provide counseling. But they should understand the emotional pain of the condition and, when necessary, help their patients find counseling elsewhere.

6. Try to determine how busy the physician's practice is. Some doctors spread themselves too thin and are too busy to answer questions, explain procedures, or respond sensitively to their patients.

We have two physicians actively involved with us. My gynecologist is a caring person but not very supportive emotionally, not particularly accessible, and gives us minimal communication. He tries, but appears very busy and is not terribly open. The urologist is never available for questions. His wife is an R.N. in the office and makes attempts at being warm but gets very defensive with questioning. I was told initially that I could see the doctor at any time for questions, but now am told to make an appointment (six weeks waiting time and $60). That's very irritating when I spend up to $200 each month for artificial insemination procedures that he doesn't personally do. My sense is

that the emotional and sexual sides of infertility are
much too hard for doctors to handle, so they avoid it as
much as is humanly possible.

You certainly want a doctor who has the time to provide thorough
and considerate treatment—time to explain, to discuss, to allow
questions, and to show some concern about how you're doing.

7. Arrange a consultation with any doctor you are seriously
   considering. This may sound like an expensive
   recommendation, but it will help answer some of the
   above questions and will be well worth the cost in the
   long run. When you go for this appointment, evaluate the
   following areas:

A. Entering the office
   (1) How are you greeted?
   (2) Is the office clean and comfortable?
   (3) Does the staff answer questions in a pleasant and in-
       formative manner?
   (4) Is the waiting room crowded?
   (5) If your scheduled appointment is delayed, are you no-
       tified?
   (6) Are there reading materials other than "new parent"
       magazines available?
   (7) Is your problem handled in a tactful and confidential
       manner by the office staff?

B. Meeting the doctor
   (1) Does the doctor greet you in a pleasant manner?
   (2) Are you given his or her full attention or are there
       frequent interruptions?
   (3) Is the doctor sensitive in taking your history and in-
       quiring about your concerns?
   (4) Is a careful and complete history taken?
   (5) Is the doctor able to listen?
   (6) Does he or she seem sympathetic and concerned?
   (7) Does the doctor welcome your questions and respond
       in an informative manner?
   (8) Is the doctor willing to share information about his or
       her background and practice?

(9)   Does the doctor clearly explain what is involved in an infertility investigation? Are lay terms or medical jargon used?

(10) Does the doctor's manner set you at ease?

And finally, recognize that you may be spending a considerable amount of time with the doctor you select. Choose carefully.

After two years of intensive treatment, the doctor's office had become my home away from home. I had read every magazine in the waiting room, knew the office routine like my own household, and had become closely involved with the office staff. Friendships even developed with others who had similar cycles and were seen regularly for the same appointments. Medical treatment took over my life in a way I had never suspected. There was nothing as important as that schedule of appointments, for that office was the place I felt would be the answer to my prayers.

Beginning Testing and Treatment

Taking the first step of contacting a physician means admitting to yourself that there may actually be a problem. People often go for long periods of time denying that a difficulty exists. Numerous fears about that initial appointment can surface: Will there be a specific problem and, if so, is it treatable? What kinds of sensitive questions will be asked? Will the doctor tell you that you are overreacting and that it is too early to look for difficulties? At this point and continuing on through your treatment, you will probably experience the same ambivalence over and over again. On the one hand, you wish to find a specific problem that is clear, treatable, and will bring results quickly; on the other hand, you would like to be told that there is no recognizable difficulty. The latter would mean, however, that you remain in limbo, wondering why you have had no success in becoming pregnant.

Most people are probably not prepared for the intense experience of a first appointment with an infertility specialist. It can be stressful and overwhelming. First, there will undoubtedly be a pelvic examination which is anxiety-provoking in itself. A semen analysis may also be required at this time. The doctor is likely to ask intimate questions about your sexual history and present sexual relationship. The process of the infertility evaluation will probably be explained, and you may feel bombarded by the myriad of tests to be completed. And all that is just to find out what's wrong. If treatment options are also mentioned, you may question why you ever decided to make the appointment. Physical, emotional, and financial worries can have you shaking in your chair, but try to remember that getting medical help is a wise decision.

Expectations when first seeking help tend to be very high, especially with the increasing news coverage of success stories and amazing technical advances. Then, all of a sudden, you arrive at the doctor's office and begin what is often a long process of diagnosis and an interminable period of treatment. Reality can be painful when you expect to receive a single definitive diagnosis and a rapid cure, only to find that answers are frequently not easy or clear-cut.

> *When my doctor first told me I was to have a laparoscopy, I was convinced that he would find some minor problem, correct it, and everything would be fine. Unfortunately, he didn't find anything (I know that sounds terrible) and told me I was perfectly healthy. I was just to keep trying. I wanted to jump out the window. I still can't accept this as it is now five years that we've been "trying."*

Sometimes what begins as one problem slowly escalates into a myriad of other factors contributing to your infertility. It can be a frustrating and anxiety-provoking experience.

During the first few appointments, try to familiarize yourself with the office so that communication in the future will be easier. Find out the names of nurses or other staff members with whom you will be in contact. Also, question what days and hours the doctor has appointments and whether there is a specific time set aside for telephone contacts of a nonemergency nature. Don't be bashful— you will probably need this information sooner than you think.

Effective Communication with Your Physician

Do you sometimes feel at a loss for words in talking with your doctor?

Do you worry that you're taking up too much of his or her time?

Do you feel frustrated at not getting the information you want?

Talking to a physician is frequently not a comfortable task. There is a tendency to view doctors as godlike figures whose actions and opinions are not to be questioned. They are the experts—and you may feel you are only a dependent, unknowledgeable patient. How easy it is to feel overwhelmed and intimidated, paralyzed by the thought that any question you ask will sound naive or stupid. The anxiety of the situation, too, can often cause more confusion than not, especially when listening to medical jargon. How often have you pretended to understand what a physician is explaining, when actually it sounded like Greek? Even those who consider themselves as intelligent, successful, assertive people in other areas of life may find themselves suddenly childlike and passive in the midst of the medical profession.

It is helpful to prepare ahead of time before visiting your doctor. Compile a list of questions or concerns so that if anxiety causes your mind to go blank, you have the security of a list on which to fall back. Remember that asking questions is not only your right as a patient but a necessity in staying well informed. Try not to bombard the physician with questions, however, before he or she has an opportunity to examine you or study your records.

As you are receiving explanations or instructions, immediately repeat what the doctor has stated. That helps keep the information glued in your mind and tells the doctor whether you have understood correctly. It is also reasonable to write down answers to your questions. If an explanation is unclear, do not hesitate to ask for clarification. This is especially true if medical terminology is being used and you don't understand it. A statement such as "Could you please explain that again without the technical words? I don't understand" should suffice. If your doctor is giving instructions that seem vague, don't risk misinterpreting them; ask for specifics. It is helpful to have some knowledge about your body and reproduction, but it is part of your physician's responsibility to interpret adequately what is occurring. Also, keep in mind how often questions and concerns seem to crop up on the trip home or in the middle of the night following an appointment. Most physicians will suggest that you call if you have other serious concerns, but if they don't, ask about the procedure for further inquiry.

It is beneficial to attend appointments as a couple, especially for the initial consultation or when testing and treatment results are to be explained. If this is impossible or you are a single person, it may be helpful to have a friend or relative accompany you for moral support. It is not unusual, when under stress, to forget conversations or misinterpret what has been said. The mind plays tricks during anxiety-ridden experiences, so another set of ears can be advantageous. Some people find that using a small tape recorder can also be useful.

Normal gynecological examinations can be embarrassing and jittery experiences, but when combined with the delicate issues of infertility, such procedures become even more emotionally intrusive. When you become aware of your intense anxiety, you may chastise yourself for not remaining calm enough to understand explanations being given. But anxiety in a doctor's office is normal and it is the physician's responsibility to take this into account. Don't be unduly hard on yourself. If you find that you are exceptionally anxious and unable to "hear" what the doctor is explaining, don't be afraid to say so. He or she may offer you some time to calm down, suggest another appointment to discuss the situation, or recommend that you return with your spouse. At least, you won't be embarrassed by not remembering everything.

Ask your doctor for copies of laboratory work or any other significant reports while you are undergoing treatment. It is helpful to keep your own file at home in case you decide later to have a consultation with another doctor or in the event that you pursue another form of treatment such as in vitro fertilization.

Recognize that it is extremely important to be *active* in your treatment. It is imperative that patients learn to speak up—to question, evaluate, discuss—if treatment is to proceed well. Have enough confidence to say what's on your mind, to trust your feelings, and to judge the situation. Of course, physicians are more knowledgeable than you are in their field, but that does not mean that you must be a silent, passive participant. If you are frightened of addressing your doctor, or simply are in awe of him or her, you will be doing yourself a serious disservice.

Infertility requires that the doctor and patient work as a team in order to be most effective. No one knows your body as well as you do. Your awareness of its functioning is important so that any symptoms you experience can be conveyed to the physician. Moreover, even the best of physicians may occasionally be lax in managing a case, so you must stay on top of all testing and treatment. This is particularly true when treatment becomes long and involved, as often happens with infertility patients. Always read, listen, question, and talk with others who are in the same predicament. Being as informed as possible is not only an asset to your treatment but promotes a greater sense of control that tends to be sorely lacking during the infertility process.

> *My first doctor was a nice man but, surprisingly, he became annoyed when I began reading about infertility and especially after I joined RESOLVE. I guess I became too smart for his liking, and he was threatened by my questions and newfound knowledge. He would have been a far better doctor if he could have come down into the real world and stopped perceiving himself as a know-it-all.*

You have a right to question any action that is to occur in your treatment, but once you and your doctor have decided on a course of action, it is important that you follow through with instructions given. Also, try to express your questions or thoughts in a clear, concise manner—no one likes to listen to long-winded, rambling speeches. Sometimes it helps to practice saying what you want ahead of time.

Your requests for information should be handled in a pleasant manner. If you are hostile, always confronting, or just generally disagreeable, nobody in the office is likely to be cooperative. A little tact and courteous behavior go a long way. Remember that there is a world of difference between being assertive and aggressive. Making a request in a quiet but firm manner will bring much more effective results than a loud, demanding encounter.

As difficult as it may be, try to voice any concerns about your medical care, especially if they are significant and impeding treatment. Some physicians handle matters in a way that they perceive as beneficial to the patient, not recognizing the negative impact. For example, a doctor may not provide full information regarding an infertility diagnosis or prognosis because of a wish not to alarm the patient. In such instances, you should inform the physician of your need to have complete knowledge of what is occurring. Remember, too, that some patients don't really want to receive a great deal of information—they prefer to know only the general facts and leave the rest to the doctor. If you feel otherwise, and I hope that you do, then make that known from the beginning and, if necessary, repeat it. You always have the right to go elsewhere if difficulties arise, but it helps to discuss problems when they happen, rather than letting them fester.

Try to understand that infertility treatment can be frustrating for the physician as well as for you. Doctors define themselves as healers and do not like failure any more than you do. Some physicians may, out of their own frustration or pressure from the patient, subtly blame the patient for lack of success. They might suggest that your anger is compounding the problem and that you need to relax. This kind of comment shows a lack of insight regarding the effects of infertility and gives a clue to the physician's frustration. On the other hand, you must try not to project your own anger onto the doctor. Make an effort to recognize when your feelings are out of control and you are dumping them on the physician.

Don't be hesitant along the way to ask your doctor for a realistic assessment of your chances for achieving pregnancy. This information is crucial in considering alternatives and planning a schedule regarding treatment. If you are thinking of stopping, let your doctor know how you are feeling. He or she may be able to help you evaluate your decision.

A Checklist for Communicating with Your Doctor

1. Come prepared. Write down your questions before you arrive at the office.
2. Repeat any important points the doctor has told you.
3. Consider writing down this information.
4. Ask for clarification when necessary.
5. Attend appointments with your spouse if testing or treatment results are being presented.
6. If you are extremely anxious and having trouble hearing explanations, say so.
7. Be assertive in your requests, not aggressive.

8. Be concise in expressing concerns or asking questions.
9. Practice what you want to say ahead of time.
10. Let your doctor know if something about your medical care or the office practice is consistently upsetting you.
11. Be active in your treatment. Ask questions and stay informed.

Drugs and Surgery: What You Need to Know

Since infertility patients are commonly treated with medication and surgery, it is important to address specifically communication in these areas. The tendency of those experiencing infertility is to accept such treatments blindly with little awareness of what is happening. The desire for a baby is so strong that people will often do anything to reach that goal. This is not to say that you shouldn't pursue the available treatments, only that you should do so knowledgeably with your eyes wide open.

For example, your doctor has just recommended that you begin taking the drug Parlodel because of a high prolactin level. Instead of quickly responding, "Sure, that sounds great!" ask the following questions:

1. How is this problem contributing to your infertility, and what will this drug do to help the problem?
2. What are the possible side effects?
3. How long are you expected to be on the medication? Are there any time limits on recommended use?
4. When must the drug be taken and under what conditions (e.g., before or after meals)?
5. What happens if the medication (or the present dosage) does not have the expected positive effect?
6. Is there any problem with taking this drug along with other medications?

In addition, some of the drugs used in the treatment of infertility are potent and need to be carefully monitored. Discuss with your doctor how monitoring will occur and if there are any problems for which you should be on the lookout. You also will want to know how much experience your physician has had with the medication being prescribed, for example, some doctors are quite experienced and comfortable with the use of Pergonal, whereas others may have limited knowledge (especially if infertility is not their primary field).

Elective surgery is another common procedure during infertility. Again, there are numerous questions you should ask:

1. Why is surgery being recommended?
2. What will it accomplish? What is the success rate?
3. Are there any alternative ways of producing the same results?
4. What precisely will be done?
5. How much experience has your doctor had with this procedure?
6. What are the risks of the surgery? How often do complications occur?
7. What can you expect to happen after the surgery: what will be the length of your stay in the hospital, the length of recuperation time, the amount of discomfort, the limitations on activity?

Any type of surgery, no matter how minor, may be frightening. It is important to have all questions thoroughly answered. A laparoscopy may be no big deal to the doctor, but it probably will be to you so don't settle for cursory or vague responses.

If you have any doubts whatsoever, feel free to obtain a second opinion. In many instances, there may be multiple ways to address a problem. You need to have all the facts to make an informed decision.

The Relationship with Your Doctor during the Holidays

As we discussed in an earlier chapter, holidays are an exceedingly difficult time to manage when experiencing infertility. This stress increases, though, when your medical needs coincide with holidays and/or your physician's vacations. What a sinking feeling can develop with the recognition that you will probably be ovulating on Christmas Day and that an insemination is needed. In addition, you may come to rely very strongly on your doctor and those regular appointments for support and sustenance throughout treatment. To learn that your physician is taking a vacation may lead to feelings of abandonment and a sense of desperation that you cannot manage on your own. Even if medical coverage is sufficient, the physician should recognize the power a patient invests in him or her and the dependency that develops. Obviously, doctors have every right (and need) to take a vacation, and holidays come whether you want them to or not, but at least the doctor should understand the patient's feelings.

How do you handle these situations? First of all, doctors ought to inform their infertility patients of upcoming vacations and any substitute coverage. If the problem is a holiday that interferes with treatment, you should be aware of this possibility ahead of time (if your cycle is at all predictable) and discuss the dilemma with your doctor. Panic at the last minute is uncomfortable for everyone. Many infertility specialists make a concerted effort to meet with a patient, even around holidays, when there is a special need (as with an insemination). Often, an arrangement can be made with other staff at your doctor's hospital or with the person covering the practice. If you are using donor insemination, it is crucial to schedule this ahead when the need will coincide with a holiday. Timing may not be precise, but if you are determined not to miss a cycle, some treatment is better than none. If medications are being used, discuss the plan for the month ahead with your physician, including how to handle various predicaments (e.g., whether you should have a second HCG injection if your temperature does not rise as expected). Not everything is predictable, but the better informed you are, the less likely you will become panic-stricken by the unavailability of your doctor.

The issue of how treatment is handled over holidays or vacations is something that can be raised early in your contact with a physician. How a doctor responds to the question should give you an idea of how much help is provided when that circumstance arises. Remember, too, that it is always possible for you to decide to skip a month and take a short vacation yourself, even though many consider this to be an unwelcome alternative.

When to Change Physicians

One of the most difficult decisions in the infertility process can occur when you consider changing your physician, especially if you have had a long-term relationship with that person. There is no question that it is easier to change doctors early on rather than waiting until treatment has continued for months or years. That is why it is so important to choose carefully in the beginning and closely examine the qualities of the person you have selected.

The following points should be taken into consideration:

1. How prompt is your doctor? It is comforting to know that your physician has a successful, busy practice, but your having to wait an hour or more for the majority of your appointments is a nuisance and a sign of poor office management. Understandably, an infertility specialist must often schedule patients at the last minute because of erratic menstrual cycles or emergencies, but this is a component of the practice and must be anticipated by the physician. To overschedule constantly because a practice is excessively large or to schedule too many patients into a short time period would be an irritation to anyone but is especially stressful to infertility patients who are already bombarded by pressure.

2. How accessible is your physician? How quickly does he or she return telephone calls? Are they returned at all? You should recognize that doctors have numerous demands on their time and that you are not the only patient. However, it is reasonable to expect that your calls will be returned and, one hopes, not days later.

3. How much expertise does your physician really have in infertility? Although this individual may have a passing interest in the field, has the doctor had experience with a large number of infertility cases and is or he or she up to date on the newest research and treatments?

When I first moved to this area, I picked someone out of the phone book who said he specialized in infertility. I was crying as I talked to him on the first visit, and he was very uncomfortable with that. He didn't allow me to express my feelings. I then got a referral from RESOLVE but didn't take their suggestion to go to an endocrinologist, rather than a general gynecologist. I figured I had a simple problem, and that I'd be embarrassed to go to a specialist with something that could be easily fixed. So I made my own choice. In spite of getting all my testing done quickly, this second

physician ended up missing a subtle ovulatory problem.
I finally switched to an infertility endocrinologist who
diagnosed my problem. After all this, I feel that any
couple with infertility should go to a specialist who has
been recommended rather than working with the local
gynecologist. But I know that it was hard for me to
make that step—it meant really facing my problem.

4. Does your doctor explain the procedures that you are undergoing, and how clear is the explanation? Does he or she encourage questions and seem responsive to them? It is very important for infertility patients to understand their situation. Increasing your knowledge of infertility and reproduction is an excellent way to establish some sense of control over your life. A physician who seems offended by your questions or who is patronizing ("Don't worry yourself. I'll take care of the situation. There's no need for you to know") should be avoided. Technical explanations filled with medical jargon and clearly beyond a patient's understanding can also be a means of keeping you in the dark. They may be used to impress you or to keep you at a distance. Neither reason is valid.

5. How available is your doctor for tests and treatment on those days when the office is normally not open? It would be wonderful if you could schedule your cycle to fit conveniently into your life and the doctor's available hours, but obviously you cannot. Ovulation has a remarkable way of occurring on weekends, holidays, and at other inconvenient times.

The greatest thing about my doctor has been his
availability. I've been going through donor
inseminations and it always seems like ovulation
comes at the wrong time. I panic every month that I
won't be able to be seen at the right moment, but my
doctor has always come through. If he's going to be out
of town, he arranges for another doctor to see me. And,
when necessary, he has even met me at the office on a
Saturday afternoon or Sunday night. It's a wonderful
feeling to know that everything will go well.

6. How aware is your doctor of the emotional aspects of infer-

tility? Has he or she ever asked how you are managing to cope with the many stresses of this problem?

> *I adore my doctor and have the utmost confidence in him. He is very thorough and always willing to talk to me. Once I left his office quite upset, feeling rotten, and later that day he* personally *called me to see how I was doing.*

7. How sensitive is the doctor's staff to the issues of infertility? A nurse or secretary must be aware of the panic you might experience when your temperature rises unexpectedly on "day 9" or when it is "day 22" and there has still been no change. Also, staff who openly and loudly discuss pregnancies and deliveries show an insensitivity to the infertile patient.

> *When my ob/gyn referred us to an infertility specialist, we were pleased with the doctor, but found that he had a staff of the most insensitive people you could ever meet. They were cold and abrupt, treating people as if they were machines. There was absolutely no awareness of the problems we were facing. After a few months, we just stopped going there because it had become unbearable. It's really a shame because the doctor was okay.*

8. How often do you find yourself in a waiting room full of pregnant women? Although this cannot always be avoided, physicians who carry both an infertility and general ob/gyn practice should have different hours for the two groups. It is excruciating for most to sit in an office surrounded by pregnant women and babies on a regular basis. Doctors should also have reading materials in their office other than parenting or "new mother" magazines.

9. How involved is your doctor with your particular case? Does he or she think about your treatment plan at any point other than the few minutes with you at appointment time and provide a sense of direction regarding future efforts? Physicians have many patients and cannot be expected to remain on top of all cases at all times nor to remember all the details of a particular situation, but there should

be a general treatment plan in mind. It may be helpful for you to remind your doctor of significant aspects of your case and to ask pertinent questions about the future ("I've been on Clomid for almost a year now. Do you think that a change to a different medication, such as Pergonal, might help?"). Even if your question shows a lack of clear medical understanding, it conveys your interest in pursuing treatment further. Physicians should be receptive to this questioning and open to discussion.

10. Finally, does your physician convey a sense of respect for you?

Remember that you always have the option of seeking a second opinion, which does not necessarily imply a change of physician. The field of medicine, and especially infertility, is not an exact science wherein diagnoses are always precise and treatments are clearcut. Various doctors have different points of view or different ways of handling the same situation, and they vary enormously in their experience and expertise. No physician worth having will object to your obtaining a consultation or a second opinion. Don't be afraid you will make him or her angry. Many people worry that they will upset their doctor and cause him to provide less efficient care; in reality, though, the request for a second opinion will probably put a doctor more on his toes. Depending on the circumstances, you might say: "We understand your point of view about the need for surgery but would feel more comfortable having a second opinion" or "It seems like you've done everything possible to help us conceive, but before stopping treatment, we'd like to hear if anyone else has another idea."

Getting a second opinion may be especially indicated if (1) either husband or wife has not been thoroughly evaluated (e.g., a postcoital test for the male is not sufficient); (2) there is a recommendation for major surgery; (3) there appears to be some withholding of information; or (4) drug treatment has been administered for a long time without other tests or regular monitoring. Throughout the infertility process, it is important to maintain your own set of records regarding tests and treatment. You have a right to review all such results, including X rays and laboratory work. When obtaining a second opinion, it is not necessary to have all tests readministered, provided you have previous results in hand.

Changing physicians, on the other hand, can be a very difficult experience and may promote a sense of moving backwards. Many don't do this when they should because they feel that looking for another doctor will require too much time and energy, and they cannot tolerate the idea of having to get comfortable with someone else. It also means coming to grips with the failure and lost time spent with the first physician. If complaints and concerns about your doctor are a regular issue for you, however, it may be best to move on. Infertility in itself is stressful enough. It need not be compounded by concerns regarding your medical care. If you have had a long relationship with your doctor, I recommend that you share your reasons for leaving. Not only does that force you to assess your previous treatment, but it also provides much needed feedback for the physician. What you say depends entirely on the specific aspects of your treatment, but try to state both the positive and negative points of your care. For example, you might say the following:

> *This is a very difficult decision, but I feel that it's necessary to change doctors at this point. Your practice is extremely busy and I have found, as my treatment has become more complicated, that I need a doctor who is more accessible. It's important for me to see someone who has more time to explain what is happening and who has greater availability for appointments. We've missed several months during the past year because I've ovulated on weekends and your office hasn't been open to do inseminations. I'm also not able any longer to spend an hour or two waiting each time for an appointment. I appreciate all your help and feel that your evaluation was carefully done, but changing doctors seems to be the best decision for me.*

If you do decide to switch physicians, don't make an impulsive decision or leave in the midst of an angry outburst. Think it through carefully. Evaluate the experience you have just been through so that you will be able to choose your next physician more wisely.

Remember that no doctor will be perfect and able to fulfill all your needs and demands. But there are many who do a very effective job of trying.

My physician has helped and educated me. He is very up-to-date and takes the time to keep me well informed. He communicates well with me and I know he cares. Regardless of what happens, he will be a good friend for life.

Both my ob/gyn and infertility specialist are godsends. They both have open ears, minds, and hearts. I can always get in touch with them or with their nurses, who are super. They listen and are knowledgeable about anything I have questions about. When I have an appointment, they never rush me. If there is something I do not fully understand, they both go over it again and simplify the hard parts. I feel lucky to have them.

Suggestions to Physicians

Although people sometimes fantasize that their physicians are super-human, most recognize that their doctors are not miracle workers. When infertility patients become upset with their physicians, it is usually not because of failure to produce a pregnancy. Rather, it is because of how they, the patients, or their cases are being handled—for example, with lack of respect, inaccessibility, poor communication, or lack of emotional support.

The following are some suggestions for physicians:

1. Recognize that infertility involves two people and should be treated with the participation of both partners, regardless of who has the medical problem. Attending appointments as a couple tends to bolster confidence in asking questions and expressing needs. It also increases the likelihood of clear communication.

2. It is crucial for you to be in contact with any other physician involved with the infertility treatment of the couple, so that your efforts are coordinated. It is very difficult for a couple to be caught in the middle between two physicians who are following different treatment plans.

3. Establish a testing and treatment plan with both members of the couple present. They can then discuss all pertinent issues—the order in which testing will occur, options for treatment (including

the pros and cons of each), the prognosis, the costs of the procedures, and the time schedule.

4. Be open to a patient's desire for a second opinion or suggest
it yourself if you feel there is a need for advice.

5. Develop some knowledge of the emotional aspects of infertility so you can take a holistic approach to your patient. The more
insight you have regarding the feelings surrounding infertility, the
greater your understanding of the emotional responses you are likely
to encounter. It is helpful and calming when a physician can assist a
couple to recognize the normal emotional stages of infertility.

6. Explain thoroughly, in advance, whatever procedures you
will be doing and tell the patient what to expect. It also helps to
make step-by-step comments during the test or treatment, if possible. Try to remember that what is routine for you may be a frightening experience for the patient. That blocked fallopian tube is not just
another few hours of surgery for the person experiencing it.

*After slightly less than a year without using birth
control, I went to my gynecologist to discuss the fact
that I wasn't getting pregnant. He ordered a postcoital
test as a beginning point. When I arrived that morning,
he had assigned me to an intern who proceeded to take
the cervical mucous. When he examined it, he looked at
me with a puzzled expression and asked me if I was
sure I had had intercourse that morning. (Of course, I
was sure!) I asked why and he said that he couldn't see
any sperm or maybe there were some and they were all
dead. He wasn't sure at all. I was so devastated that I
couldn't even ask questions. I wanted to crawl under
the table and cry. Fortunately, my husband and I moved
to a different state after that and I never saw that
doctor again. It took a long time for me to want to
continue the investigation. I'm sure this intern did not
realize the emotional impact his confusion and
expression of his findings had upon me.*

7. Welcome inquiries and respond to them in an understanding,
nonpatronizing manner. Even if you have just finished explaining a

point, the patient may have been too anxious to really hear you, or you may have given an unclear message. Remember that the self-esteem of infertility patients may be shaky, and they are often hesitant to ask questions for fear of appearing stupid.

8. Be honest in presenting your findings and observations. There is a value in being hopeful, but be careful that you don't convey false optimism.

9. Meet with the patient or the couple in your office during the initial appointment or when testing and treatment issues are being presented. It is very difficult for a patient to feel competent and mature when undressed, in stirrups, or sitting on a table in an examining room.

10. Be accessible. It is advantageous if a member of your office staff, trained as a nurse or nurse practitioner, is available to respond quickly to telephone inquiries. This person can screen calls to determine who really needs to speak with the physician and whose needs can be met by the nursing staff. It makes a difference to your patients to receive prompt, courteous replies, and very often calls require only a brief response.

11. Work closely with a professional who specializes in infertility counseling so that you can make referrals readily when patients are struggling with the many emotional issues of infertility. Some physicians find it helpful to have a counselor on their staff.

12. Be cautious in your use of humor. It needs to be handled carefully in treating infertility patients because it can easily be misinterpreted. Try to take your cues from your patients. If the patient often jokes and seems to use humor as a way to handle the pain of infertility, then this may be a comfortable way of relating and helping that individual to relax. Otherwise, be careful.

13. Be aware of and sensitive to the physical discomfort that accompanies a number of the infertility tests and treatments.

When I had each of my three hysterosalpingograms, the female radiologist proceeded slowly and sensitively. She explained precisely what was happening and asked if I was in too much pain. Whenever I flinched, she would notice and say, "I'm sorry that had to hurt." Her acknowledgement of my discomfort made it much more bearable.

When a physician ignores or tries to make light of the pain, the patient can feel childish, embarrassed, or angry.

14. Be familiar with RESOLVE or other local support groups and mention them as a resource to your patients.

15. Recognize your own limitations as a physician. Be willing to face the issue of ending your efforts. It is wonderful for doctors to be encouraging, especially if there is something to be encouraged about. But after a long period of infertility treatment, monthly efforts at optimism ("I bet that this will be the month!") can grate on a patient's nerves. It is hard for both patients and physicians to admit that "enough is enough," but this has to be faced, especially when patients' lives are deteriorating from the unending stress.

Patients, of course, vary greatly in the length of time they are willing and able to endure treatment, but you must be sensitive enough to note their responses and not push treatment beyond their wish to continue and their ability to cope. If the likelihood of producing biological children is not promising, gently suggest they explore alternative means of having children. It is difficult for everyone to accept failure when so much time, effort, and money have been invested, but continuing indefinitely can take a heavy toll.

Infertility and Employment

Grieving on the Job

> *My heart is just not in my work at all any longer and I don't care to do as good a job as I should. It used to be such an important part of my life, but I can't make myself feel that way now.*

Many people find that job satisfaction markedly decreases when facing infertility. Why does this happen? For some of you, the depression over infertility may become an all-pervasive feeling, expanding into all areas of your life, including your work. Feeling a sense of failure at producing a child can easily mushroom into judging yourself a failure in the workplace, too. In addition, the experience of struggling to have a child can dramatically change priorities. The career that once was so important may now seem insignificant or less rewarding by comparison.

Leaving the pain of infertility at home is hard to do.

> *There are so many times when I'm still brushing away the morning tears as I walk into my office building. I try to plaster on a phony smile, but the tears are still damp on my cheeks. In general, being at work is a relief because it's something I enjoy and it helps to keep my mind off infertility. But trying to keep that private part of me from intruding is an endless battle.*

Because feelings are often so close to the surface during infertility, it can be difficult to control them at work.

170

I am now trying to get some self-control, but until recently I found myself getting snappy with people, feeling irritated at the least provocation, and ready to burst into tears at any conflict. You could look at me cross-eyed and I'd feel my eyes start to well up with tears. I don't feel that my personal problem should interfere with my job or that I should take out my feelings on others, but it's been hard to stop.

Those with jobs that relate, in some way, to their infertility situation, such as obstetrical or pediatric nurses, or teachers, may find it exceptionally painful. Many find that they eventually have to leave jobs that are too emotionally demanding or that strike too close to home.

I used to work as a counselor in the child-adolescent unit of a mental health center—a job I loved. During one year I was there, however, I had eight adolescent clients who unexpectedly became pregnant and decided to have abortions. I struggled painfully to deal with this, as it was my job to help them arrive at a decision and work through their choice. Even though I believed in free choice to have an abortion, it was a constant fight inside myself to stay objective. My own issues kept interfering, although I'm sure I hid it well. Handling my anger at their ease in getting pregnant and my constant failure was so hard. It felt like a slap in the face.

I work at home as a day care provider (stupid job for an infertile person!). I began doing this work right after we were married because we were going to have kids right away and I wanted to be home with them. Obviously, things didn't work out that way. Working with preschoolers and infants is very hard, although it's not so bad now. I used to resent them. I had thought of quitting numerous times, but this is what I want to do and I'm good at it. There are still some days when I don't want to face a bunch of wide-eyed little people, but the good seems to outweigh the bad.

For people who have delayed efforts to have a family in order to establish a career, managing an infertility problem and managing work can be particularly troublesome. These individuals tend to be very goal oriented, striving for success and often attaining it. To suddenly find themselves with a goal that is out of their control can have a great impact on their approach to life and their career. Infertility is a startling blow to anyone, but especially to those who are high achievers and have come to believe that any objective can be obtained through hard work and perseverance. When they realize that this isn't always so, it is not unusual for their work performance to decline suddenly and for their involvement in their career to diminish. An assumption about life and themselves has been shattered.

Handling Career Decisions

Indecision is likely to plague all areas of your life when you are experiencing infertility, but it can be especially evident and detrimental with employment issues. People often postpone decisions about their work because they believe that they might be pregnant the next month.

> *Three years ago I was in a very dissatisfying job and suddenly a new opportunity became available. At the time, my husband and I were just beginning our efforts to conceive and I assumed that it would be a matter of a few months before we were successful. I agonized over the decision, questioning how I would handle pregnancy and work. I almost didn't take the position, but then decided it was too important to pass up. Thank goodness, I did. My husband and I are still waiting for that child. As miserable as infertility has been, at least I've had a job that makes me feel good.*

> *On three occasions, an interview for a promotion was available at my job. At each time, though, I was depressed about my infertility and didn't feel like applying for the promotion. Now it's hopeless. I guess I'll now just have to stay at my position without any advancements.*

It is certainly difficult to think about a career when your world is confused and your future uncertain. Trying to evaluate your feelings about work can also present many questions.

> *The stress level on my job is quite high and the politics of the administration results in low morale and rapid burnout. I burnt out approximately two years ago, but at that time the job stress and lack of satisfaction was not a concern. My husband and I had planned to start our family. With this in mind, I was not worried, as my pregnancy would be my key to freedom. I had no idea that conception was going to be a problem. Now, I am not sure whether to start sending out résumés. I am confused as to whether my lack of motivation at work means I am no longer interested in my chosen career. My uncertainty about my future ability to conceive makes it difficult to make any career plans. Do I assume that my job dissatisfaction means that I should prepare for another career? Does the constant uneasiness relate to my infertility? What if I decide to go back to school and then become pregnant? These questions and subsequent anxiety over the answers have immobilized me. Instead of doing something, I've become unable to do anything regarding my career. I keep hoping that someone will come up with a magical answer.*

As this woman suspects, there are no magical answers because everyone's needs are different and no one can foresee the future. The following questions, however, may help you to evaluate your feelings and needs regarding a career decision.

1. Did your job dissatisfaction precede your infertility problem or has it developed in the midst of tests and treatment?
2. What originally made you choose your present career? Are those reasons still valid or important to you?
3. How important is having a career?
4. Despite any dissatisfaction in your position or at your place of employment, are there aspects that are rewarding?

5. How flexible is your present job regarding your infertility treatment? Does its location create difficulties with regard to keeping regular medical appointments?

6. Can you presently handle the stress of a change—moving to a new position or a new place of employment, returning to school, switching careers? Would a change cause you to fall apart or would it bring a sigh of relief, perhaps a burst of motivation?

Work satisfaction can deteriorate when your personal life is so unhappy. But if your career is at all important or rewarding to you, try to continue pursuing your goals without dwelling on "what if?" Even if having a family is more important to you, infertility treatment can sometimes be a long haul. The worst that might happen is making a career move and then finding it impossible to complete because of pregnancy. How bad can that be?

Coping with Co-Workers

My office seems to average about one delivery every month and, of course, there is a party for every one of them. My co-workers seem to delight in decorating with pink and blue for the parties and buying the most adorable gift you can imagine. It's bad enough having to watch bellies grow on a daily basis, but the parties are devastating. I want work to be a haven from my personal problems—however, it's become anything but. The worst part is the comments from unknowing others who always kid, "Hey, I bet you'll be next." Don't I wish!

Whether or not you choose to tell co-workers of your problem must be a personal decision. Some find it helpful, discovering tremendous support and understanding.

I work in a medical setting and found it necessary to tell my boss and some co-workers because of my frequent doctor appointments and because of the precautions necessary for pregnant women being in contact with certain diseases. The people I work with

are very special people, and they adapt readily to my
appointment schedule or are willing to take a patient
during those times when I'm questioning pregnancy. I
feel guilty for all the time I take, though, particularly
since it cannot be well planned for.

I am an R.N. in the labor/delivery department, so it has
often been difficult for me to see babies being born
every day except to me! About six months ago was the
first time I informed any of my co-workers what I was
going through. Once they knew of my problem, they
were very helpful and supportive. Somebody is always
coming up to me with a new miracle treatment. Also,
now that we're hoping to adopt, I have half of the
hospital looking for a baby for me.

On the other hand, many feel that their colleagues would not be
sympathetic, and they see no advantage in sharing their predicament.
Some worry that any disclosure of their efforts to become pregnant
would either harm their chances of a promotion ("After all, if I never
get pregnant, I might as well have the opportunity to move up the
ladder") or reflect badly on their emotional capacity for handling the
job ("I don't want anyone at work to know how much I'm struggling
with this problem. It makes me feel weak, as if I should be able to
handle it better").

It does help, though, to have at least one close friend at work
who is aware of and sensitive to your infertility and to whom you
can turn when circumstances get rough. Since medical appointments
often occur on weekdays during work hours, there will invariably be
medical crises or disappointments that happen at times when you
can't escape. There may be no choice but to return to work and face
the responsibilities there. Having a close friend available with whom
to share your misery can be comforting.

There were times that I'd return to work from a
disastrous medical appointment, like having a
sonogram and finding I'd never ovulated after 21 amps
of Pergonal, and would feel like death warmed over. I'd
go through the rest of the day in a fog, almost
oblivious to my actions. I guess the motions were so

*ingrained in me that I carried it off okay, but it's a
wonder how I ever functioned! The only person at work
who really knew what was happening was my office
mate. Sometimes I just needed a few minutes to cry on
her shoulder before facing the rest of the day.*

Unquestionably, it helps tremendously to have co-workers who
are supportive and understanding. Moreover, it may also be difficult
not to let a boss or other staff members know of your problem if
medical appointments are constantly interfering with job responsibilities.

Balancing Schedules

How do you manage to keep a job *and* take off the time necessary
for medical tests and treatment? The answer to this question depends on the type of job you have and your position. People find
many different ways to balance their schedules, but usually not
without a significant amount of anxiety.

*As a sales representative, I'm constantly on the road, so
it's not too difficult to sneak off to doctors'
appointments—although there have been some close
calls. I've chosen to keep the problem to myself which
has generally worked out, except for the time I was
hospitalized for surgery. Then I made it sound more
like a female problem with endometriosis rather than
infertility. I don't know what I'd do if I didn't have so
much freedom in being out of the office.*

*I work for a large corporation and, fortunately, have
never had a problem with taking time off. My manager
and close co-workers are aware of my situation and
quite supportive. Because of this flexibility, I feel very
lucky and try not to let my concerns about infertility
interfere with the quality of work I do. Some people
here may question my comings and goings, but the
ones who really count know what's going on.*

It is important to plan ahead if at all possible. For example, if you know that the time from day 10 to day 18 is always crammed full of medical appointments and sudden shifts in scheduling, that is *not* the time to plan an important sales conference or some other significant event at your job. Of course it depends on how much control you have, but try to keep medical days as free or as flexible as possible. Many crises can be avoided if you think ahead. The tighter your schedule is during those mid-cycle days, the more stress you are certain to experience.

Many physicians have evening or weekend hours. If your job has little or no flexibility, this could be a major factor in choosing your doctor. You certainly would not want to select one who has limited hours for appointments and excessively long waits. Look, too, for a physician who is located near your job. Appointments in the early morning, late afternoon, or at lunchtime may then be possible with little disruption of your work schedule. If scheduling around work is a primary concern, make sure that you raise this issue with any doctor you are seriously considering before making a commitment to treatment.

In some cases, however, the balancing act between work and doctor appointments cannot be maintained. It may be necessary to establish priorities if wrestling with career and medical demands become too conflicting.

I essentially gave up my career. I was really moving up and enjoyed what I was doing, but the constant "shleps" to the doctor at all hours were impossible. It wasn't fair to my job and it wasn't fair to me—the stress became too much. I knew I had to do something, though, to keep myself occupied, so I went to work part time at an old job where people knew of my problem and were very supportive. But, after awhile, even that became too much for me and I eventually had to quit completely.

When I first learned of my infertility, my job was a savior. I loved it and my responsibilities took my mind off the issues of infertility. As time progressed, though, the medical demands grew and my patience waned. I found myself, for the first time, unable to sleep at night, preoccupied with concerns over infertility and work. I finally realized after weeks of exhaustion that

something had to give before I did. I felt I was on the
brink of a nervous breakdown and that was terrifying.
My career had always been extremely important to me,
but I began to recognize that infertility was requiring
an almost full-time commitment and that this, for now,
was my first priority. Fortunately, with the
understanding of my superiors, I was able to decrease
my hours to a part-time position. It was a hard
adjustment to make but an absolutely necessary one.

Some people, then, when faced with time-consuming treatments or emotional overload, are able to arrange a part-time schedule. This may be a helpful compromise if you feel unable to give up either career or infertility efforts. Another possibility, if financial pressures are not a major factor, is to take a temporary leave of absence. In considering this, however, ask yourself how you will feel without the daily structure of a job. As one woman said, "I wasn't thrilled with my job, but working gave me a reason to get up and make myself look presentable each morning." You must also consider whether your job has the benefit of insurance coverage. How good has the coverage been and will you be able to afford the premium on your own? Only you can weigh all the factors in making such a significant decision.

Evaluating the Stress of Your Job

The atmosphere and responsibilities of jobs vary immensely; some jobs are more stressful than others. It may help to examine your work situation and assess how you interact with it. For example, some people enjoy the hectic pace of a fast-moving, high-powered job and, during infertility, find that it helps them cope by giving them forty hours a week of thinking about other matters besides pregnancy. They feel alive and vibrant, instead of discouraged and depressed. For others, the stress of this sort job may be too much, especially when compounded by the demands of infertility. The same goes for a laid-back, slower paced job. This may be exactly what some people need, whereas others would find that it gives them an overabundance of time to contemplate their worries.

Since infertility is a condition that causes you to feel out of control, you may be in trouble if your job creates the same feeling.

Assess what you have control over in your work situation and what you don't. Step back a little and take an objective look at what your position entails:

1. What were you initially hired to do?
2. What other responsibilities have you taken on?
3. How much flexibility can there realistically be?
4. Is the job what you thought it would be?
5. Do you get a sense of pleasure or satisfaction from it?
6. Are you in any way creating more stress at your job than there need be?
7. Do you enjoy the people you must work with?
8. Is traveling to and from your job a source of stress?
9. Is it necessary to keep your position for financial reasons?
10. Is your job essential for career advancement?

Answering these questions can help you determine whether your job is a plus or a minus in your life right now.

Nobody knows you as well as you do. Just as you may have a sixth sense in recognizing that your car is not operating right because of your familiarity in driving it every day, such is the case with yourself. Listen to your body and monitor how you are responding to stress before it gets out of hand. You may not be able to decide exactly how much stress comes from work and how much from infertility, but you can get a general notion of its source. Sometimes people blame their jobs for difficulties in conception, assuming that the pressure of long hours, multiple responsibilities, and anxiety on the job have caused the infertility. They probably haven't, but they probably haven't helped either.

The focus in this chapter has been on the conflicts surrounding employment, as they affect women and infertility treatment. Remember, however, that for some of you, work *can* offer an opportunity to improve your self-esteem and keep from feeling like a total failure. As one person said, it can be a very "normalizing" experience in the midst of feeling different and alone.

For the moment, infertility has destroyed my homemaker aspirations, but it has made me establish a very stable, profitable career which I enjoy and keeps me busy. It also has helped to enhance the material quality of our lives. Had children come along quickly and easily, I doubt that I would have been as motivated to pursue my career.

Conditions of Special Concern

Secondary Infertility

Barbara and Jack have a beautiful six-year-old daughter, conceived shortly after their marriage. It had been an unexpected pregnancy and came at a time of financial instability. Although they were delighted with their child, they quickly began using contraceptives in order to prevent another surprise. They wanted to be ready, emotionally and financially, the next time. Several years passed, and now, they were prepared for a second child, excitedly looking forward to expanding their family. Everything was "right" this time, except month after month went by and there was no pregnancy. Initially they were bewildered—it had happened so easily the first time. But feelings of frustration and failure grew. In desperation, they made an appointment with an infertility specialist.

This is not an atypical story. Just because you have been able to get pregnant once does not necessarily mean that you will be able to conceive easily again. In fact, one government study found that, of all infertile couples, 60 percent are facing problems with secondary infertility—a condition suffered by those who have had a biological child but are now unable to give birth to another baby.[1]

The causes can include any of the factors that contribute to primary infertility. It is possible that a physical problem has developed since the birth of the earlier child or that a previous difficulty (most likely unknown at the time) has grown more severe. Whatever the reason, the success rates for overcoming primary and secondary infertility are similar.[2]

Reacting to the Crisis

Those of you who are experiencing secondary infertility problems will have many feelings in common with other infertile people, such as anger, guilt, and depression. The pain of learning about others' pregnancies and births will probably be just as devastating. But this condition has some unique characteristics. These people can feel caught between two worlds, fertile and infertile. Because others are skeptical about their infertility, they may be less sympathetic. They cannot understand the tension and sadness that pervade your life when they see that you already have a child. All the disturbing comments made to infertile couples are heard, too, by those with secondary infertility. But in this case, someone may add, "Well, you've had one baby; you should feel grateful for that." This comment suggests that the couple has no reason to be upset.

Joining a network like RESOLVE, a tremendous support for many infertile couples, may create a dilemma for those experiencing infertility the second time around; they may ask, "Do we belong?" To gain support and acceptance from other infertile people, those of you with secondary infertility may find yourselves almost apologizing for your previous success and then feeling guilty over this deemphasis of your present parenthood. You may worry that others in RESOLVE will feel angry or resentful of your presence and, in some cases, that may unfortunately be true.

People with only one child may be subject to intrusive inquiries regarding their "decision": "Oh, you have just the one child?" The assumption is that having a single child has been a choice or that the conception occurred by accident. Others may jump to the conclusion that you never really wanted children at all. On the other hand, some expect that you want to expand your family and wonder what is taking you so long. They may even attribute selfish motives to your one-child situation, assuming you do not want the aggravation of more children or are reluctant to lose free time.

Those with secondary infertility can feel frustrated and bewildered over the problem, having succeeded earlier. Some may deny the possibility of infertility and delay efforts at treatment. Even after having sought medical help, the denial can still exist.

Guilt is another common emotion experienced by those with secondary infertility—guilt for not being satisfied with the child they have, guilt for being depressed and bitter toward others, and guilt for not being able to provide their child with siblings. Just as couples with primary infertility question their lives to determine what mistakes they made to warrant their condition, the couple with secondary infertility may search for the reasons they deserve to have only one child. Because they were able to conceive before only increases their guilt; they imagine that they must have done something wrong to be afflicted with infertility now.

Effects on the Family

The emotional turmoil and the stress of infertility treatment can have an impact on your child. If you are feeling depressed or angry, you may convey these feelings to those around you, withdrawing from your child or becoming easily irritated by minor annoyances.

> *Sometimes I can't function and I feel like a lousy mother and a worse wife. The last two weeks of my cycle are murder on me, my son, my husband, and my friends. I've been lucky to have friends who, for the most part, have been supportive. But my daily functioning has suffered, my house goes without cleaning for days, and my appearance is not to be believed.*

A child may also become worried over your emotional state, especially if you cry a great deal. You should explain to the child, in terms appropriate to his age, that he is not responsible for your unhappiness. Children often blame themselves for their parents' difficulties.

Your youngster may add to the pressure by asking, "How come I don't have a brother or sister?"

> *My five-year old daughter asks when she will have a brother or sister. I can only explain that I can't have any more children. She doesn't really understand, and I believe she thinks that I mean I "won't," not "can't."*

> *My child has wanted a baby since he was two years old. He is now the only five-year-old who knows about*

*hormones, how to make babies, and why Mommy cries
when the doctor calls. At four, he wanted to know,
"What can I do to help you get pregnant?" That's when
I briefly told him about sex. After my miscarriage, he
wanted to know why the doctor couldn't go home and
look up in his book why the baby died, so it couldn't
happen again. He goes with me for my Pergonal shots
and has asked the nurse to teach him "so Mommy
doesn't have to come here." We had karyotyping done
and he learned about chromosomes. When the phone
call came that the chromosomes were good, he
responded that now "we" could get pregnant. How
many kids think that mommies have to get shots to be
able to get pregnant?*

*How many have to live in a home full of stress
and depression, having to hear that Mommy is very
tired, has a headache, or is very sad? He is extremely
compassionate and loving, trying to understand what is
happening, but it is not fair to him or me. We are
missing out on a lot together. He is picked on too much
and yelled at too often for reasons that could have
been avoided. I have been trying to make a conscious
effort to laugh more with him, spend time together, and
to hug and cuddle him. I don't want to waste his
childhood over a baby that may never come.*

Your child may also be faced with questions from his friends as
to his only-child status. It can be particularly worrisome to deal with
a young child who pleads for a sibling and cannot understand why
he can't have one. Some children may feel that you are deliberately
depriving them of a brother or sister. They may even fantasize that
they are at fault, that their "bad" behavior has led to their parents'
refusal to have more children. An older child might question why his
parents are so unhappy and struggling so hard to have another baby:
he may think "Aren't I good enough?" It is such a confusing and
overwhelming time for an adult that one can hardly expect a child
to understand. But you should try to rectify any serious misconceptions.

Some of you too, can fear that you will lose your only child through illness or accident and then translate this worry into over-protection. You may also expect perfection from the child, fearing there will be no other offspring to fulfill your dreams.

Coping with Secondary Infertility

The frustrated desire for another child can be exacerbated by a lack of support and understanding from friends and family. In coping with this problem, first recognize that you have a real and legitimate concern. Don't be hesitant to get medical help after a year of unsuccessful efforts to conceive. Others may tell you to "just relax," but a medical opinion is in order.

In struggling through secondary infertility, it helps to communicate with others who are enduring a similar experience. Some RE-SOLVE chapters have support groups specifically for those with this problem; if they do not, they can put you in contact with other members, for chapters keep lists of people with specific infertility problems. Having the opportunity to share your frustrations with someone who understands can be very beneficial.

Since you do have at least one child to care for, you must recognize the impact of the problem on him, in terms of the emotional reaction you convey to the child and the effects on him of having no siblings. Your upset over infertility is understandable, but you mustn't let it destroy your relationship with your child. Savor your time with him. If you find yourself unable to give emotionally to your child because of despair over infertility, seek help through a support group or a counselor.

Too often the negative side of having an only child is emphasized, yet there are many positive aspects worth considering. Studies have shown that marital satisfaction lessens as the number of children increases, even when comparing families with only one or two offspring. Enjoyment as a parent also diminishes as a family gets larger.[3] Only children tend to receive more attention than those with siblings, including time, money, and affection. Educational opportunities are also greater for the only child and achievement levels are often high. Although the desire for another baby can be strong and you may decide to go to great lengths to have a larger family, it might be helpful to remember there are advantages in having just one child.

Pregnancy Loss

> *As I write this I am pregnant for a fifth time. My first*
> *four pregnancies ended in miscarriage. I have told only*
> *a few people, nearly all of them friends from RESOLVE. I*
> *know I cannot bear to hear people say, "Oh, how*
> *wonderful! Congratulations!" It is impossible to*
> *convey to most of them that no, it is not wonderful, at*
> *least not at this point; that being pregnant is*
> *frightening and anxiety producing, and a situation in*
> *which daily life feels like walking on eggs. My husband*
> *and I talk rarely about this baby and we don't really*
> *allow ourselves to think of "it" as a baby yet, even. I*
> *am superstitious, procrastinating, in a state of*
> *emotional neutrality. I am merely waiting. It is not a*
> *pregnancy celebrated and enjoyed like other women's*
> *pregnancies. Yet way, deep down, there is a very secret,*
> *very private place where all the self-protective, insulting*
> *behavior does not seem to penetrate. Tiny, light-filled*
> *fantasy images scamper out for whole minutes at a*
> *time before they are ruthlessly squelched and shoved*
> *back inside the dark recesses of safety. ("Will she have a*
> *funny, lopsided smile like her father's?" "Will I nurse*
> *him here by this window?") Hope is always there, in*
> *little glimmers, impossible to deny. Yet, like a general*
> *marshaling huge armies, I ward off, fortify against*
> *those feelings. When and only when I hold that baby in*
> *my arms, will I allow myself to feel that pent-up*
> *explosion of joy.[4]*

Losing a pregnancy can be a highly painful experience, and, as
this woman's poignant account makes clear, the effects may be long-
lasting. If pregnancy loss has happened once, one often fears it will
happen again. It is a cruel experience, allowing a flash of hope and
excitement, only to lose it all suddenly. For those who have struggled through months of infertility, it is rubbing salt in an already
painful wound.

A miscarriage, one form of pregnancy loss, refers to the premature delivery of a fetus that is unable to survive on its own. In
medical terminology, it is more accurately labeled a "spontaneous

abortion," but the more familiar term will be used here. You may be surprised to learn that an average of one out of every six pregnancies ends in miscarriage.[5] That percentage increases with the woman's age, from 12 percent at age twenty to 41 percent at age forty-two.[6] That amounts to approximately 300,000 miscarriages yearly in the United States, and added to the number are those people who have to endure ectopic pregnancies, stillbirths, or loss of a newborn.[7]

What Causes a Pregnancy Loss?

Causes of pregnancy loss are numerous, including chromosomal abnormalities, hormonal problems, structural difficulties (an abnormally shaped uterus, a double uterus and vaginal tract, large fibroid tumors affecting the interuterine space), and immunological problems. Most miscarriages are caused by chromosomal abnormalities. This does not necessarily indicate a genetic problem in the parents. Rather, it tends to be a chance circumstance in which an abnormal fetus is developing and is naturally aborted. Thus, the majority of miscarriages during the first trimester are unavoidable because the fetus probably would not otherwise mature beyond the three-month point. Seventy-five percent of miscarriages do take place during the first trimester, with the remaining 25 percent occurring from twelve to twenty-four weeks.[8] Beyond this time, the loss of a baby is considered a stillbirth.

Initial Reactions to the Loss

When bleeding occurs during a pregnancy, anxiety will skyrocket, as the couple worries over the likelihood of the baby's survival. Often, this will be accompanied by a feeling of helplessness, especially when a physician offers no advice except bed rest. Even though miscarriage is usually not a life-or-death situation for the mother, the symptoms of bleeding and cramping can intensify with heavy blood loss and severe contractions. It can be both frightening and painful, and the sense of being out of control will surely escalate at this time. Not uncommonly, the woman suffers from a state of shock, especially if the pregnancy loss occurs quickly and without warning. One minute, she is overjoyed with the prospect of a baby and the next, she's in despair. "It must be a nightmare," she thinks. "I'll wake up and everything will be all right." But it isn't. For many, a state of numbness persists as they grapple with the painful reality.

Other fears are common at this time. Many worry that a hysterectomy will be needed, but this is rarely necessary. Others may panic, believing that a miscarriage automatically implies that they will never be able to have children. The fact is that a single miscarriage means only that that particular baby has been lost, unless medical evidence reveals some persistent problem.

At the time of the miscarriage, it is especially important that medical staff be sensitive to the physical and emotional crises that are occurring. It helps tremendously if doctors explain what is happening and give careful instructions.

> *My doctor knew I was bleeding, cramping, and would probably miscarry, but neglected to tell me to save some of the fetal material for tests. I was very angry when asked after the fact if I'd saved it. At such a painful time, I did not think of saving it but would have done so if the doctor had so instructed.*

Many couples also complain that they were not given emotional support throughout this time. Concern over the physical effects of a miscarriage usually outweigh attention to its emotional impact. Medical personnel may be uncomfortable with death and use distance or rigid composure to handle their feelings. Or they may be so used to miscarriage they have grown immune to their feelings and fail to recognize the traumatic effect on the couple. Physicians are often quick to provide medication for the woman in an effort to calm her and "make her feel better." But she and her husband need the opportunity to grieve. Watching this can be distressing for an onlooker, but it's important to the couple. Sensitive and compassionate medical staff can be a tremendous help to them.

> *When we lost our baby, both of us became hysterical in the hospital. I'm sure it looked like we were going crazy, and there were probably some who were ready to admit us to the psychiatric ward. Fortunately, our doctor understood our need to carry on like this even if others didn't. I realize now just how important it was to let out our grief, and I feel sorry for those who are forced to swallow it.*

Unfortunately, treatment often occurs on or near the maternity or obstetrical unit. It doesn't take much imagination to recognize how upsetting this can be—to experience the pain of loss while watching others joy. If you are hospitalized during a pregnancy loss and the only option is care on an obstetrical floor, ask your doctor for a room with some privacy, apart from new mothers and babies. It can also be helpful to request that your husband be allowed twenty-four-hour access to the hospital under such circumstances. It is a time when husbands and wives need to be together.

Institutional care can hinder the grieving process, and medical centers and their staff need to develop more sensitive means of handling these painful situations.

The loss of a much wanted baby is not an easy thing to forget. I remember how happy we were during those wonderful days when we knew I was finally pregnant. My doctor arrived at the hospital in muddy boots and dirty jeans, muttered "She's going to abort," and left. Shortly afterwards, I was sent home without anything to numb the physical or mental pain. I was told to return to the hospital when I began to pass tissue. It was all so hard to deal with, especially because our baby was so planned, so wanted. Also, I ended up next door to the delivery room where a woman was delivering her baby. It seemed as if no one cared about our loss. It is experiences like this that disillusion, hurt, anger, and cause me to lose all faith in the medical profession.

Comments made by medical personnel can sometimes also be insensitive or inappropriate.

I have had at least five miscarriages, and most people act as if it is no big deal. One doctor said, "Oh, it was only a zygote." That was the baby I had waited over five years for. That was years of D-and-Cs, semen analyses, chromosome tests, blood tests, basal body temperatures, X rays, and more. It was not "only a zygote." The other stupid comment is "You weren't that far along." I've been "expecting" for over five years. How would most people feel if they lost a five-year pregnancy?

*When I miscarried, the doctor and resident I saw were
compassionate, and the nurse brought me a warm
blanket. She did make a few very inappropriate
comments, however. She said she always told women in
these situations something that was probably difficult to
hear which was that it was probably all for the best.
Then she told me to think of the fun of trying again.
Trying to get pregnant again is never fun for an
infertile person. It seems to me that if this nurse was
aware of her comments upsetting other women, then it
was her professional responsibility to examine whether
her comments were insensitive.*

Most people who hear such comments are surprised and
tongue-tied, unable to express their anger. It would help, however, to
let medical staff know of their inaccurate or insensitive remarks.
Your comments need not be made angrily, but they should reflect
your distress: "I know your remark was based on medical facts, but
when you've been through years of frustration with infertility, a
miscarriage means a lot more than that. It's a baby that we've struggled for, and what you said made us feel worse." Inaccurate remarks
like "Think how much fun you'll have trying again," should definitely
be addressed. Without feedback from patients, medical personnel
will continue to be unaware of the impact of their statements.

How deeply you feel the pain of a pregnancy loss will depend
on several factors. If you lose a baby after a long period of efforts to
conceive, you will experience the loss differently from someone
who was not planning a pregnancy.

*My first miscarriage was very early—just a few days
after learning I was pregnant—and not too long after
we'd first tried to conceive. To tell you the truth, I was
just happy to have conceived. I know it sounds crazy,
but even to be pregnant for a brief time made me
hopeful. But not so with the second miscarriage. It was
two years later and I was three months pregnant, when
a sonogram showed trouble. Even before the results
were clear, I was in tears, completely devastated. My
husband just lay next to me on the bed with his arms*

around me for the rest of the afternoon. What was
worse was that I had to spend Christmas weekend
waiting for a miscarriage. It was horrible—I wouldn't
talk to or see anyone. My family fortunately came over
and made me talk to them. Eventually, with time, I got
over it. But it took a lot of time.

Other factors affecting the intensity of grief will include whether you have other children, your history of previous miscarriages, your age, the suddenness of the event, and how far your pregnancy had progressed.

On one extreme, some people are so devastated by the experience that they fear its recurrence and avoid efforts to conceive again. Others quickly swallow their feelings of sadness and immediately resume trying to get pregnant, avoiding the much needed time for healthy grieving. The crucial point here is that grieving is appropriate and necessary, regardless of how long the baby was in utero. Even when the miscarriage has occurred early in the pregnancy, the loss may be very real. Falling in love with the child can begin the moment a positive pregnancy test result is received. Don't feel you're overreacting if you are upset over a miscarriage that occurs during the first few weeks.

Coping with the Loss

Just as there are no rituals for the monthly grieving an infertile woman experiences with the onset of her period, there are also no specific aids for working through a pregnancy loss. What is more, there is nothing tangible to mourn. As Tim Page wrote in a poignant article, "Life Miscarried":

It is not merely the numbing, animal sense of loss that
causes us to flinch from the subject; it is the abstract
quality of that pain. For an unborn child could be
anything at all: it is ours, it is us, but we know little
more. We can only imagine the color of its eyes, the
chime of its laughter, the breadth of its dreams. There is
nothing concrete to mourn, only a negation of infinite
possibility.[9]

During the recovery period, most will feel a great sense of emptiness. For a while, though, the reality of the loss may not sink in and there will be continued fantasies of pregnancy, especially with the lingering physical signs of breast tenderness and a distended belly. It is not unusual now for the person to pretend—to deny what has happened and to hope, childlike, that the nightmare will go away.

Despite the tenuous nature of the loss, it is critical to acknowledge it and face up to the intensity of the feelings. Grieving cannot be sidestepped by pretending the pregnancy never occurred or by rationalizing the miscarriage ("Everything happens for the best"); nor should you rush back into activity to erase the painful feelings. The process of mourning is best helped by remembering what has happened and talking or writing about the details of the pregnancy and miscarriage.

Failing to resolve the loss can have serious future repercussions. It could develop into a full-fledged clinical depression or inhibit bonding to a baby in a later pregnancy because of the fear that this baby, too, will not survive. Failure to mourn can also negatively affect the relationship with a child you already have. Parents may develop excessively high expectations for this youngster who must "make up" for the loss of the baby.

The grief reaction after a pregnancy loss is not unlike that experienced when a loved one dies, but several elements make this process different. First, you are likely to feel intense anger which is magnified by the closeness of the loss to the joy you experienced earlier. And as in all aspects of infertility, there is that feeling of being out of control that only adds to the rage. Often, the anger will be displaced onto your obstetrician, especially if you feel, rightly or wrongly, that the physician could have done more to help prevent the loss. Sometimes, doctors can bring anger onto themselves through their own behavior. By not acknowledging the emotional impact of pregnancy loss—perhaps because of their ignorance or their uneasiness regarding the subject of death—they fail to relate to their patients on a sensitive level. Support and understanding from a physician will discourage displacement of anger and can open the doors to helping patients effectively handle their loss.

Second, you may also feel intense guilt at this time since frequently there is no specific reason for the loss. One forgets how common miscarriage is and imagines that one has been singled out for "punishment." Or you may be plagued by guilt over past trans-gressions and perceive your pregnancy loss as "God's judgment" on your sins. You may well begin dissecting your life, questioning what errors you made to cause this (Did I eat the wrong foods? Should I have gotten help in lifting those heavy groceries? Was I under too much stress at work?). When others offer suggestions for handling the next pregnancy ("I'd take it easy the next time, if I were you, and not do so much exercise"), the comments may reinforce your sense of personal failure, exacerbating the guilt.

Men, too, may experience guilt, most commonly with regard to having had sexual relations during the pregnancy, although studies have shown no correlation between miscarriage and incidence of sexual intercourse. In some cases, a husband will blame his wife, which can be a particularly destructive situation—pulling a couple apart when they desperately need each other. A simple statement by a physician—such as "Most miscarriages happen strictly as a chance event and there's no indication that you could have done anything to stop it"—can help immensely in lessening guilt and blame. Remember that physical exertion rarely causes a miscarriage, except in cases when a fetus is already defective.

Poor self-esteem, feeling less of a woman, is likely to surface now, especially when you perceive others as mastering pregnancy so easily. Being pregnant is often considered a narcissistic state with the fate of the baby closely connected to a woman's feelings about herself. Thus, an inability to nourish and sustain a baby is seen as a personal failure. A woman may feel intense anger toward her body, believing that "it" has caused the death of the baby. Herz, in "Psycho-logical Repercussions of Pregnancy Loss," says that "this split of the normal experiences of unity of mind and body, another form of turning against oneself, creates a potentially devastating conflict."[10] A woman may also feel that she has disappointed her husband and that her "failure" could cause him to leave her. These concerns should be discussed openly between husband and wife before they grow into major fears.

Social Implications

Feeling isolated and unsupported can be a major obstacle to grieving after a pregnancy loss. Many of you may be reluctant to mention the situation out of embarrassment, sadness, or guilt, and therefore, others may not be aware of your pain. Even when friends or family know about the loss, they may not consider it to be a significant event or a reason for distress. People are quick to relate to the pain experienced in the death of a loved one, but too often there is little understanding of the despair over pregnancy loss, particularly miscarriage. Others may even seem indifferent. Even if they accept your grief, they usually do not realize that grieving takes time. They want to hear only that you are coping well and quickly getting back into the swing of things. Expectations from others for rapid recuperation, especially from one's husband, can be a major strain.

Often, friends or relatives will shy away, not only because they don't know what to say, but also because they fear their presence might be unwanted. They may be waiting for you to say something. Try taking the first step by letting others know that you want and need their support. It seems unfair for the burden to fall on you, but the reality is that most people are ill prepared for handling another's loss.

Also remember the many other people who have experienced miscarriages and may be able to relate to your pain. They can be a source of support and confirm that your feelings are normal. Women who have positive relationships with their mothers might find understanding by sharing their feelings with them.

You must protect yourself now from painful experiences, for you are very vulnerable. Be kind to yourself. When a loved one dies and people are in mourning, they are not expected to attend joyous social events. The same is true for you who are grieving after a pregnancy loss: you do not have to attend a christening, a birthday party, or some other celebration. If the guest of honor is a special friend, speak to her about your feelings and find some other way to let her know you care. If the relationship is not a close one, you might offer a reasonable excuse for not attending and then send a small memento of some sort.

It can be especially difficult if a friend is experiencing a successful pregnancy. Coming to terms with why her baby is growing and yours died is heart-wrenching. Unfortunately, too, you may notice that other pregnant women shy away from you after miscarriage. They do not believe in a rational sense that your condition is "catching," but many women fear miscarriage and your experience makes their fear all too real.

The Husband's Role

Pregnancy loss is an emotional crisis for both men and women. But often it is the husband who must be the "strong" one, the wife's "protector," and he is not given the opportunity to grieve himself. It can be emotionally painful to be the person who can only sit help-lessly, watching someone else suffer. Many men, when given the chance, talk of how frightened they were when their wife miscarried and how upsetting it was not to be able to do anything.

Husbands often don't know what to say; they are overwhelmed by their emotions and a sense that they should somehow "make things better." They will frequently conceal their feelings for fear of upsetting their partner further. They believe that they must be strong to keep their wife from falling apart. Sometimes, men will put on a mask of cheerfulness in an effort to drive the painful feelings away or they will become extremely busy, encouraging their wife to do the same. This is usually not helpful, though. Most women want to know that their husbands share in the hurt, and both of them need time to face their loss. It may be beneficial to lessen responsi-bilities and social engagements for a while. Providing mutual comfort can be an important step toward healing.

One should understand, however, that men and women do have different ways of handling their grief and that there is no "correct" behavior in responding to loss. The woman, rather than focusing on the differences and feeling angry that her husband is not reacting as she is, should be aware that he is feeling and expressing his grief in his own way. She should remember, too, that because she is the one who carried the child, her reactions may understandably be more intense.

"How Long Will I Feel this Way?"

Working through the pain of pregnancy loss will not be accom-plished overnight. Depressed feelings can linger for weeks or months and it is not unusual for interest in sex, especially on the part of the woman, to vanish during this period of depression. As grieving pro-ceeds, however, the pain will recede, and eventually you can accept your loss. Suddenly, you may realize that you aren't crying any longer and that you are again able to enjoy your previous interests. Of course, the emotional struggle with infertility may continue to plague you.

Even when you feel that you have successfully handled the situation, periods of grief may recur long after, especially at significant "reminder points" (the onset of menstruation, the anniversary of conception or of the miscarriage, the expected time of the baby's delivery). If you let yourself fully grieve, however, these anniversary reactions will ultimately stop. The memories of the loss will not disappear, but the intensity of feeling will gradually diminish.

Early Hysterectomy

A hysterectomy refers to the surgical removal of the uterus, including the cervix. When one or both tubes and ovaries are also removed, it is called a hysterectomy with salpingo-oophorectomy. A hysterectomy, under any circumstances, can be an emotional experience but an early hysterectomy, occurring before a woman has had children or before a couple has fulfilled their expectations for a "complete" family, is a significant blow.

The surgery may be the necessary course of treatment for any number of conditions, including cancer of the uterus or cervix, extensive fibroid tumors that have not responded to drug treatment and seem inoperable, severe endometriosis causing intense pain, uncontrolled infection, or severe uterine hemorrhaging. Endometriosis is now one of the most common reasons women in the United States have hysterectomies, although many physicians consider this to be an inadequate reason. Physicians usually make every effort to save the uterus and ovaries in women still wanting or waiting to have babies, but, sadly, this is not always an option.

Reacting to a Hysterectomy

Emergency hysterectomies in a young woman are not frequent but when they occur, they can be exceptionally hard to handle because there is no emotional preparation time. On occasion, it may be a life-or-death situation, in which case the initial concern is only to protect the patient's life, not to worry about loss of her reproductive organs. This, unfortunately, may impede the grieving process, especially if the woman is told that she should feel grateful to be alive.

Even if the surgery has been performed electively because of severe pain or abnormal bleeding, and the operation brings relief of these symptoms, adjustment can still be extremely difficult. This is especially true, of course, for those who have not had children and are longing for them. It may be somewhat easier if the woman has known of her infertility for a long time and efforts at treating the problem have been unsuccessful. But grieving is *always* necessary.

The grieving process is not unlike that for pregnancy loss or other aspects of infertility. Apart from the reality of not being able to bear children, however, there is the added misery of losing part of your body. The uterus symbolizes the woman's ability to have children and, for many, it is the essence of being a woman. Its removal means no longer menstruating and no longer having the hope of becoming pregnant. Some women say they do not see themselves as female, or more commonly, that they feel "less of a woman."

There is a great deal of misinformation on the subject of hysterectomies. Everybody knows somebody who has had one, and they may confidently relate, in an authoritative manner, their ideas of how a hysterectomy will affect your life. The belief of women "going crazy" from having a hysterectomy obviously is an old wives' tale, although depression is not uncommon and grieving should be expected, especially in the case of a childless woman. But no studies have indicated a causal relationship between hysterectomy and severe mental problems, except in those instances where the woman already had a history of or predisposition to such a disorder.

"Will a Hysterectomy Affect Me Sexually?"

Many women worry about the effects of this surgery on sexual functioning. In the recent past, women were told that there would be no change in sexual response. Masters and Johnson once stated: "A woman will be as sexually responsive after her hysterectomy as she was before she developed the symptoms . . . for which the surgery was performed."[11] In other words, those who never enjoyed sex in the past were unlikely to enjoy it after, whereas those who did find pleasure would continue to do so. The only exception was for those who previously experienced pain in making love because of problems that led to the hysterectomy. For those women, sex might now become more comfortable.

Masters and Johnson, however, are now recognizing the significance of uterine contractions in orgasm. For many women, then, there may be a change in sexual response that is physically, not psychologically, based because of the absence of these contractions following a hysterectomy.[12] This does not mean that these women are no longer interested in or responsive to sex—only that their response may be different. Honeycutt, though, in his book *All about Hysterectomy*, notes that some women who previously experienced uterine contractions continue to feel a similar sensation, despite the fact that the uterus is gone.[13] On a rare occasion, a woman will complain that she misses the feeling of the man's penis striking against her uterus but, for most, this was probably never a pleasurable experience.

Effects on the Marital Relationship

Many women worry about how their husband will respond to them, believing that the surgery has made them "different." A woman may fear that her partner will no longer find her attractive or feminine, or that, because this clinches the infertility diagnosis, he will now want to seek another woman.

Often, the worry exists that the hysterectomy will cause an accelerated aging process. But, a woman's appearance or desirability will not be altered by this surgery unless she causes it to happen. How people think they will change after a hysterectomy can sometimes become a self-fulfilling prophecy. It is not that a hysterectomy causes a person to become "fat" or "old," but rather that a preconceived idea and a poor self-image can unconsciously create this situation.

Although most men are supportive and able to work through their feelings about their wife's hysterectomy and her inability to bear children, some may feel resentful and cheated. Once aware of these feelings, they may then feel guilty for having them. It is important that the husband who feels this way discuss his feelings with a physician, counselor, or men's support group.

The Response of Others

Dealing with the fertile world after a hysterectomy can also be difficult. Perhaps the most typical response by others is the remark, "Well, at least you don't have to put up with periods anymore!" Again, others often mean well but are either ignorant or insensitive to the deep meaning of the loss. Many will make such comments in an attempt to deny the pain of the experience, always looking for a "bright" side. It's not that they don't care; it's only that they are uncomfortable and don't know what to say. All the usual reminders of infertility (babies, showers, birthday parties) will apply equally in this situation, but there are others that may be just as painful—friends complaining about their periods or advertisements for tampons and sanitary napkins.

Handling inappropriate remarks is never easy. You can always give a brief response like "Believe me, I'd give anything to have my period again," which at least lets people know that their comment was wrong. If you want to pursue the issue further, you can explain how you really feel. With particularly offensive people, it helps to turn the tables and ask the insensitive person how she would feel if her uterus was removed and she couldn't have children. Chances are the conversation will end abruptly.

Recurring Doubts

It is not at all unusual for a woman to question the need for the hysterectomy in the years afterward. Therefore, the more positive you feel about its urgency at the time it occurs, the less tormented you will probably feel later. Unless the hysterectomy is necessary in an emergency situation, you should always try to obtain a second opinion. Spouses must also openly discuss the surgery and its implications before proceeding if it is done electively.

DES Exposure

The drug DES, short for diethylstilbestrol, was a synthetic estrogen developed in 1931 and first administered to women in 1945 for the purpose of increasing chances of a successful pregnancy. It was often given to pregnant women with a history of repeated miscarriages or in situations where diabetes, toxemia, or premature delivery seemed to threaten the pregnancy. For many years, DES was considered a safe drug and was administered to millions of women, especially during the late 1940s and 1950s. Its use was continued until 1971 when studies began to reveal that females who had been exposed to the drug in utero were later showing an increased incidence of vaginal cancer. Some reports have indicated that as many as 5 million individuals, including pregnant women and their offspring, were in contact with the drug during those years.[14]

During the 1970s, studies also began to reveal that exposure to DES in utero could lead to structural abnormalities in the reproductive system, affecting both women and men. It has been found that in women the anatomical effects usually involve the uterus, cervix, and fallopian tubes. Because of these abnormalities, a common plight for the DES daughter is repeated miscarriages, although it should be noted that with each successive pregnancy, there seems to be an increased chance of successful completion. "Slightly more difficulty in conceiving" has also been indicated.[15] With regard to the male, some studies have indicated a possible correlation between DES exposure in utero and an increased incidence of defects in sperm analysis (low sperm counts, poor motility, abnormal structure).[16] Some exposed men have also been found to have abnormally small testicles. It is ironic that a drug once used to preserve pregnancy is now being linked to reproductive failure.

Many women initially became concerned about their DES exposure because of worries that it might be carcinogenic, only to learn later of possible additional effects on their fertility. Others recognized the potential hazards of the drug at the point of trying to conceive. The problem of DES exposure is especially disconcerting because the victims have been reaching reproductive age only in recent years and available information is still sparse and uncertain. Obviously, it can be very frightening to be afflicted with a virtually unknown condition. This, again, intensifies one's feelings of being out of control.

Emotional Responses to DES Exposure

Infertility that is DES-related can have serious emotional consequences for both the infertile patient and the mother who took the drug. Both may be intensely angry, and often that anger is projected at the treating physician or the medical profession in general. This is probably a displacement of rage felt toward the mother's obstetrician who prescribed the medication.

My mother had five miscarriages before the doctor gave

her DES for me. I knew I had an increased chance of spontaneous abortions, but I thought the doctors would be of more help. I've already had five miscarriages in five years. Why couldn't the doctors have helped me based on my mother's medical history? I am angry because a lot of my suffering could have been prevented if doctors were more knowledgeable.

My anger is very difficult to handle because I know it is often irrational. I can usually talk myself out of depression by counting my blessings, but it is hard to talk myself out of anger. I feel anger at my husband, friends, family, and strangers; anger at the entire medical profession; anger at parents who don't appreciate their children; anger at people who have abortions; and yes—anger at God. By suppressing all this anger, I find myself releasing it at the most inappropriate times. I get angry at the silliest things which most people would ignore.

The effects on the mother-daughter relationship (little has been studied regarding the emotional effects on sons) seem to vary significantly, based on the status of the relationship prior to learning of the DES-related infertility problem. If mother and daughter have had a caring relationship, chances are that this crisis will produce improved communication and a sympathetic bond. If, however, there has always been tension or negative feelings between the two, the situation is likely to exacerbate the previous problems.

Guilt tends to be the overriding feeling on the part of the DES mother, and it is common for her to become very involved in her daughter's infertility treatment. Some daughters, though, become reluctant to speak with their mothers for fear of intensifying their mother's feelings of guilt or worry.

The Doctor-Patient Relationship

Apfel and Fisher, in the book *Infertility—Medical, Emotional, and Social Considerations*, note that physicians are likely to minimize the extent of emotional distress involved with DES exposure.[17] This can create much difficulty. How the physician reveals findings regarding DES and how he or she relates to the patient are crucial in this situation. Physicians must appreciate the impact of what they are saying, being careful to present the facts in an open and honest manner with realistic discussion and clear explanation. They should be cautious, however, not to alarm the patient with technical and confusing jargon. Sensitivity on the part of the doctor is the key. Without that, physicians may elicit even more anger from the patient.

Patients and their doctors must also work together in evaluating and treating the problem. Women (or men) are likely to be easily angered or offended by a physician who takes a paternalistic stance, saying "There's nothing to worry about. I'll take care of everything." The DES patient has had firsthand experience with the fallibility of the medical profession and will probably not regard such an authoritarian stance in a positive light. Doctors also need to understand that owing to the unknown factors involved in the previous use of DES, many DES offspring are reluctant to take any medications that might have a deleterious effect on themselves or potential children. Mistrust can be very strong.

Getting Help

The sense of aloneness associated with infertility is especially strong in the case of individuals with special types of infertility problems. Both DES mothers and children need support and help in working through their feelings and in recognizing that their predicament is not an unusual one. A group such as DES Action can be very helpful in providing newsletters and support groups to those facing DES issues. There are two national offices to contact: (1) Long Island Jewish Medical Center, New Hyde Park, NY 11040, and (2) 2845 24th Street, San Francisco, CA 94110.

For pamphlets that provide information on DES-related cancer and other concerns, write to Office of Cancer Communications, National Cancer Institute, Room 10A17, National Institutes of Health, Bethesda, MD 20014.

The High
Technology of
Parenthood

There used to be few options available to childless couples, but that situation is rapidly changing. Medical technology is advancing by leaps and bounds, and infertility is becoming big business. Donor insemination, in vitro fertilization, and surrogate parenting are just a few of the options now available to infertile couples.

Although these procedures bring hope (and often success) to those suffering infertility, they are not without some concern. Each carries with it a special set of questions and worries that must be tackled before choosing that particular option. And once a decision is made, there are additional stresses to be faced, unique to each procedure. Going through any of these treatments is not easy, but then nobody ever said that infertility itself is an easy experience.

The purpose of this chapter is to clarify some of these common fears and stresses so that you will be better able to assess the options for yourself. Being knowledgeable and well prepared is far preferable to rushing forward blindly, and it is essential to your emotional well-being during these experiences.

Donor Insemination

In the United States, artificial insemination by donor, AID, is increasingly being used by infertile couples with a high rate of success. It may surprise you that approximately fifteen thousand infants will be delivered this year who were conceived through AID.[1] Reports indicate that 80 percent of all women attempting to get pregnant with donor sperm will accomplish their dream within six months.[2]

Many are also unaware that artificial insemination is not a new medical procedure. It was first successfully accomplished in 1866, using husbands' sperm, and by 1890, it was being utilized with donors. Few realize the prevalence and success of this procedure because it is so rarely discussed.

What Is AID?

The procedure is used when the husband has an untreatable infertility problem, most commonly identified as azoospermia (no sperm production) or oligospermia (sperm concentration less than 20 million/cc with few motile sperm). It can also be the treatment of choice in some cases of Rh incompatibility or in the event of male genetic difficulties which the couple fears could be passed on to a child.

Medically, the procedure is simple and usually pain free. It involves obtaining semen from a donor and inserting it (fresh or thawed after being frozen) into the woman's vagina, near the cervix, by means of a syringe. Extensive research into the freezing of sperm has shown that AID with frozen sperm is safe and offers many advantages over use of fresh semen. Fertility, however, may be somewhat impaired in comparison with fresh specimens (success rates are approximately 25 percent lower for frozen semen).[3] After insemination, the woman then remains in a reclining position for twenty to thirty minutes. Sometimes a physician will put the semen in a cervical cap, which is placed over the cervix, remaining up to three hours. On average, the procedure is administered twice per month around the time of ovulation.

Selection of a Donor

One of the first questions which couples are likely to ask is, "Who is the donor and how is he selected?" That can be a tremendous worry for obvious reasons.

> *I wonder a lot about the donor but worry less now than in the beginning, especially since I'm now going to a doctor in a major city. Initially, I was using a physician in a smaller town and worried about the donors being obtained on a more casual basis through newspaper ads. It wasn't a real organized program there, whereas now the donors are very accessible*

*through a hospital program. I still hope that his nose
won't be too big or his glasses too thick—but it really
doesn't bother me as much.*

In the past, it was usual for couples to receive little information
about the donor. They might be told that some of the husband's
physical features or the couple's religion would be matched with the
donor but, in general, they had to rely on the physician and other
staff members to handle the selection in a responsible and ethical
manner. Having to place full trust in others about such an important
decision was, and still can be, frightening and awesome.

Increasingly, however, couples are beginning to request more
information, and rightfully so. As a result, they are able to have a
greater sense of control in the AID process. The following are some
questions that a couple should ask before insemination occurs:

1. Where does the semen come from (a sperm bank, a
   hospital, or the doctor's own donor program) and how did
   the donor become involved with the program?

2. What screening procedures were completed on the donor
   to assess his fertility and to insure a clear medical history?
   Some examples of screening procedures would include a
   semen analysis, semen culturing for sexually transmitted
   diseases, testing for sickle cell disease or Tay Sachs disease,
   and a complete blood profile that checks for syphilis,
   hepatitis, and other conditions. Screening for AIDS virus is
   also required in many programs. What were the results of
   the semen analysis? Are donors checked every time they
   donate? If multiple inseminations are necessary (in any one
   month or for future pregnancy attempts), will an effort be
   made to use the same donor?

3. What reasons did the donor give for wanting to donate his
   sperm?

4. What information is recorded in the chart regarding donor
   and couple?

5. What are the physical characteristics of the donor—hair
   and eye color, skin tone, race, ethnic background, blood
   type?

6. What is his educational level and his area of work or
   educational specialization?

7. Does the donor have any prominent interests or abilities, such as musical talent or athletic prowess?

Doctors and sperm bank programs vary in their ability and willingness to offer this information. If you have a desire to know these facts, arrange a consultation with your doctor before proceeding. Trying to determine a physician's policies by telephone or through office staff may not provide you with thorough information. Also, a consultation gives an opportunity to discuss all aspects of the AID procedure, both physical and emotional, in order to make an informed decision.

In regard to matching, efforts are made to match the physical characteristics of the husband and donor, including height, body build, coloring, and blood type. Religion and ethnic background can also be taken into account. Donors must be of at least average intelligence, have demonstrated fertile potential, and be screened to rule out any ill health or hereditary problems. Often, they are medical students or residents and thus are easily accessible to the physicians providing AID services. The amount of screening and the acceptibility of a donor into a program, however, will vary immensely. For example, at Idant Laboratory in New York City only 15–18 percent of those who apply are accepted as donors.

Emotional Preparation for AID

Although AID is medically a simple procedure, the emotional issues are complicated and intense. Most find that the actual experience of donor insemination is far less difficult than making the decision to follow this route. Some people are intellectually able to decide on AID, only to find later that they have neglected to face its emotional impact. Sometimes these unresolved feelings will surface unexpectedly in the future or be displaced onto other situations.

Couples must allow themselves to grieve over the loss of the biological child they thought both would bear before embarking on a course of AID. The decision to pursue donor insemination involves a mourning process of its own because it means that the dream of conception and the fantasies of parenthood must be reconsidered. It also means that there will be a certain "inequality" between the parents, which should be discussed. Conception will not result from a moment of loving sexual union, as the couple had expected. Certainly, a child conceived through AID can represent the love between spouses and their special emotional union, but the biological union will not have occurred. It is not unusual for a wife to experience as strong a sense of loss as her husband over his inability to contribute genetically to a new generation. It can be difficult to accept that the traits or characteristics of her mate that she admires so greatly may not be continued in their offspring. It is important that the couple realize that although it is the husband who is experiencing untreatable infertility, it is something for which *both* partners must grieve.

The Husband's Concerns

Although the issues surrounding the consideration of AID will be stressful for both husband and wife, they will perhaps be more intense for the husband. As in other aspects of male and female infertility, the use of donor insemination may exacerbate already existing feelings of inadequacy and poor self-esteem. Anger, on a conscious or unconscious level, is very common. Not only is the man feeling inadequate because of his infertility; he must also endure the thought of another man's sperm impregnating his wife. In some instances, a husband may equate donor insemination with adultery, failing to view the procedure strictly as a medical technique. It does not help that some religions, such as Roman Catholicism, do consider it to be a form of adulterous conduct. Adultery and AID are most likely to be irrationally equated if a man has low self-esteem or has been unable to resolve the negative feelings surrounding his infertility. A few men may carry their feelings a step further and develop a fear of their wife deserting them in favor of the donor, believing that she has fallen in love with this unknown person.

A husband may not only be disturbed by the idea of impregnation by another man's sperm but also feel left out of the whole procedure.

> *Sometimes I worry that my husband feels like a fifth wheel—totally unnecessary in the process. He initially voiced some desire to go with me for the inseminations, but my doctor was pretty negative about it. He (the doctor) just didn't feel it was necessary.*

The husband may also question the future implications of AID, for example, fearing that he will be excluded from the family, with his wife and child forming a special loving bond of which he cannot be a part. Associated with this may be doubts as to whether his wife will consider him to be the true father. In this sense, some men specifically worry that they will not be given full participation as fathers and that their opinions in raising children will not be valued. From a personal standpoint, then, the husband must ask himself many questions: "Will I be able to love this child as I would love a biological child?" "Will I feel distanced in the family or make myself into an outcast?" "Have I resolved the feelings about my infertility or will this child always remind me of my sense of deficiency?"

In some cases, a man may feel guilt ridden and consider himself selfish should he refuse AID, thus preventing his wife from carrying and delivering a child. Agreement based on guilt, however, is not wise. Uncertain feelings should be discussed openly or future trouble can be expected.

The woman has an important role in her husband's overall adjustment to the use of AID. She must be very sensitive to his feelings and help him through the difficult adjustment period of learning to accept his infertility. Although a man's sense of inadequacy may not be pervasive, especially if he has a strong self-image and is confident of other areas of strength in his life, it seems unlikely that he will not have some negative feelings. If he denies them, chances are the underlying sense of anger, frustration, or sadness will appear elsewhere in disguised form. An aware and sensitive wife can help her husband with the realistic expression of these feelings so that resolution becomes possible.

The Wife's Concerns

Emphasizing the woman's supportive role is not to say that emotional issues for the wife when considering AID will be absent. First, she may worry about the actual procedure, questioning whether it will be uncomfortable or embarrassing. It is usually not painful, although some cramping might occur, and it is no more or less embarrassing than a pelvic examination.

A woman must also deal with the fact that pregnancy will not be achieved in the "normal," perhaps romantic, way envisioned. A few women may be disturbed by the feeling that they are being physically violated when undergoing AID. Of course, being artificially inseminated is not like making love with your husband, but it does not engender the loathsome feelings of being raped. Somewhere in the midst of these experiences come the feelings stirred by the insemination process. Regardless of intense wishes for a baby and a willingness to endure just about anything, a woman may find herself uncomfortable with the act of receiving sperm from someone other than her spouse. It can be a strange experience for a woman to travel to a doctor's office each month for inseminations without her partner present. Some women may also resent the fact that they carry the bulk of responsibility in enduring this treatment, even though it is not medically "their" problem.

As a result of all these feelings, many find it comforting to have their spouse attend the appointments with them and to perhaps combine it with a special opportunity for lunch or an afternoon together. The procedure becomes somewhat more natural with both partners present. It is crucial for the man to recognize the importance of his support and participation in easing his wife's anxiety.

Like the husband, a woman too may experience anxiety regarding the future implications of AID. A frequent worry is that her husband will not have the same depth of love for the child as she does and may, at some time, become rejecting. If any physical or emotional problems develop in the child, the woman may also fear that she alone will be held responsible for these shortcomings. All these concerns need to be discussed openly between partners.

Having Sex after AID?

Many couples find it helpful to make love following an insemination. In certain cases, where the husband has a low but not absent sperm count, this may serve to blur the question of who the biological father is, should the woman become pregnant. Some find that this uncertainty is a more comfortable means of accepting AID (although it could be viewed as denial of the issue), whereas others find the ambiguity to be a greater strain. From a medical point of view, Silber in *How to Get Pregnant* states that there is a scientific basis for suggesting that some couples (when husbands have some viable sperm) have intercourse after donor insemination has occurred. Although it is unlikely that the husband's sperm will impregnate the wife, it is not an impossibility. He states that the initial donor sperm entering the cervical mucous tend to form a passageway along which others will travel. His belief is that these first sperm may die in the process, allowing others to follow toward fertilization.[4] Other physicians recommend abstaining from intercourse around the time of insemination, especially if AID efforts are not initially successful.

Some physicians make a practice of combining semen from the infertile husband and the donor to cloud the issue of biological identity. From a medical standpoint, however, this method is controversial. Some believe this lessens the effectiveness of the fertile sperm, while others feel it is worth a try for a few months before using only the donor semen.

Thoughts about the Donor

The woman having fantasies about the donor is not unusual, especially considering the many unknowns in this treatment.

I often questioned who this person was, who every month provided me with some new hope. On one occasion, when my doctor suddenly decided that I needed an extra insemination, I came to the office and had to wait for arrival of the sperm. After a long delay, a young bearded man appeared with a small bag in hand which he gave to the nurse. Shortly thereafter, I was called in. I often wondered if he was just a messenger or actually "the one."

When I started with AID, I learned that most of the donors were actually interns or residents at the hospital where I worked. Often, when I walked around the hospital, I would think, "Gee, that's a good one! I hope he's in the program."

Some may allow their fantasies to flourish and find comfort in this, whereas others may repress such thoughts in an effort to keep the process as anonymous as possible. It is also not uncommon for there to be occasional worries that somehow a mix-up has occurred and the wrong semen has been inseminated.

Becoming Pregnant with AID

Despite intense joy, anxiety is likely to skyrocket in both partners upon learning of pregnancy following AID. Panic may suddenly develop as both question their actions and wonder about the results. Before embarking on use of donor insemination, a couple's only concern may be to achieve pregnancy but, once they are successful, the underlying fears can become acutely felt: What will the baby look like? Will he have any problems physically or intellectually? How will we be as parents and how will this change our lives? These concerns are common to all prospective parents, regardless of how conception occurs, but it may be especially difficult with the many unknowns surrounding AID. Also, fears of delivering a defective baby may increase because of the nature of conception and a sense that it was "artificially" done. Those with unresolved guilt regarding the decision may be particularly afflicted with doubts. For example, some may still be experiencing religious constraints against AID, questioning whether they are going against God's will and creating a life that was not meant to be.

Those who have had a successful first experience with AID and return for repeated attempts tend to be less anxious. Most important, though, it has been found that once a pregnancy progresses, both parents are able to participate emotionally in the experience and AID does not seem to hinder a sense of love and closeness with the child. When the baby is born, there may be intense concern about who the infant looks like, again owing to the unknown aspects of the biological father. But those worries tend to be short-lived. Being able to discern features that resemble either the mother or father (even though he is not genetically responsible) can bring a sense of relief.

This may sound ridiculous, but one of my biggest fears was that our baby would be born with a full head of red hair—when we are both brunettes! How would we ever explain that? We had planned to keep the whole issue to ourselves and yet a red-haired baby would have been a major complication. Seeing a perfectly healthy, brown-haired infant brought a sigh of relief.

"Should We Keep It a Secret?"

The secrecy surrounding artificial insemination by donor is one of the most difficult aspects of this technique. Anxiety regarding disclosure may first be apparent at appointment times, as you wonder who else in the office knows about the insemination and whether any other patients saw the "AID" next to your name in the appointment book. The issues of how much information about the AID process should be shared and with whom are troublesome and need to be reflected upon carefully.

Do you tell family and friends?

If you do, will that change their feelings about you and your baby? How would you handle negative or embarrassing comments?

If not, can you handle the lifetime of secrecy?

Should your child be told of his conception?

What feelings will this produce in him, if you do, and how can you respond to the lack of information available regarding his biological father?

There are still many biases against donor insemination and couples must question the implications of these feelings for themselves and their child. The Roman Catholic church, as I have pointed out, considers AID to be a form of adultery, thus making illegitimate any children conceived in this manner.

Despite a desire eventually to handle the issue honestly with the child, this does create some difficulty. First of all, children will be incapable of understanding the meaning of artificial insemination until they have clear knowledge of reproduction and, even then, the concept of AID may be confusing to them. In addition, since insemination is not an openly discussed, commonly acknowledged procedure, it is likely to make a child feel strange. As difficult as it may be for adopted children to work through all the issues regarding their birth parents and the adoption, it would probably be even more troublesome for the AID child, owing to lack of information and minimal social supports. As one woman experiencing AID said, "I think that it would be opening up a whole can of worms that is entirely unnecessary."

Others do feel differently, however, like this man:

I had to think long and hard about how I felt about donor insemination, especially how I would feel after a child was born and was growing up. I have resolved these issues in a positive way, though, and feel good about the decision. The child, if conceived, will be told about these decisions and our experiences. It would be impossible for me not to be open and honest with a child. I'd go crazy trying to conceal it. I consider it a positive approach. It, to me, would be easier to discuss with a child than would the circumstances of an adoption, since there may be a lack of love somewhere down the line when a child is given up for adoption. There will be no lack of love here. I just hope our child, if conceived, won't be spoiled rotten.

Most couples, at this time, choose to keep the decision secret between themselves, and the majority of infertility specialists recommends this course of action. That means that friends, relatives, and other physicians (including one's pediatrician) are usually unaware of the use of AID. It can be difficult not having the opportunity to talk openly about the decision, especially when a couple feels that it is an acceptable route to take and they have no regrets about it. By shrouding the issue in secrecy, it can make the grieving process exceptionally hard because it means that you must handle the pain alone or only with your spouse. For a woman, knowing that her husband is already feeling a deep sense of loss and perhaps guilt over his "failure," there is often a reluctance to burden him with her additional grief. As a result of these factors, and in spite of the push for confidentiality, I think that it can be helpful to open up to a special trusted friend, a member of RESOLVE who has acknowledged use of AID, or a professional counselor, especially if you are experiencing some turmoil in trying to settle the emotional questions surrounding donor insemination. RESOLVE has an anonymous AID contact system available through its national office.

The Issue of Confidentiality

In order to maintain confidentiality, physicians usually use a coding system in their records regarding the couple and the donor. At times, records of the donor may even be destroyed so that all trace of the biological father is eliminated, preventing any future attempts at disclosure. This practice of record destruction is often criticized, however, by those who believe that such information should be maintained in the event that medical history is later required regarding the offspring. Others also feel strongly that a child's rights to knowledge of his biological origin are violated by this practice. Speak to your doctor regarding the procedures used in his or her practice.

Legal Implications of AID

Before concluding, a few remarks should be made regarding the legal issues associated with AID. Although this procedure has been practiced throughout the country for the last thirty years, a large number of states have no legal provisions for its use. Only twenty-five states now deal with the rights of offspring conceived through AID. Legitimacy of these offspring was first declared in the United States by the Georgia courts in 1964. There, the law states: "All children born within wedlock . . . who have been conceived by means of artificial insemination are irrebuttably presumed legitimate if both husband and wife consent in writing."[5] Other court cases have focused on the position of the husband (as opposed to the donor), clarifying his legal rights and responsibilities for the child. A 1968 case carried to the Supreme Court of California brought a landmark decision that made the consenting husband responsible for child support upon later dissolution of the marriage.[6] Further court rulings have largely been based on this precedent, providing the nongenetic father with visitation rights in situations of divorce. Offspring conceived by AID have also been provided with inheritance rights.

Consent forms should be signed by both parents once they have received a clear explanation of the insemination process. A consent form usually gives permission for the physician to perform AID, removes all responsibility from the physician or hospital regarding any potential congenital deformity, and indicates the nongenetic father's responsibility for care of the child, including financial support and inheritance rights.

Making the Decision to Use AID

The use of AID is likely to foster questions and thoughts a couple never before considered. Unfortunately, the questions far outnumber the answers. The more you think about the procedure and search for concrete assurances, the more anxious and confused you can become. Certainly, the decision to pursue AID should be carefully thought out, but at some point a couple must allow positive emotions to rule, focusing on the joy of having a baby and becoming parents. Overintellectualization of the procedure can be detrimental.

Despite this discussion of the difficult emotional issues, it must be noted that many people approach AID with few, if any, reservations. Their only concern is having a child, and they are willing to do anything to achieve that end.

> *For me, the idea of AID was never a big deal. I knew*
> *early on of my husband's sterility, and insemination*
> *never seemed like a terrible thing. We both agreed easily*
> *to pursue it and I just felt, "If it works—great!"*

Many men are able to resolve their infertility and are committed to the idea of being fathers, regardless of their lack of biological contribution. For those who are fearful of future negative effects on the marriage, it should also be noted that divorce among those with AID children is rare. One follow-up study found that only 1 in 800 marriages had resulted in divorce (as of at least seven years post-AID).[7]

For those who have relatively little apprehension about the procedure itself, the worst part of experiencing inseminations may be the inconvenience and unpredictability.

> *The most difficult aspect of AID for me is the lack of*
> *control I have over the process. The frustration of being*
> *totally dependent on the doctor, his office, the donor,*
> *whether it's a Sunday or holiday, etc., is unbearable. I*
> *really haven't had a "good" cycle in the last six months*
> *because of the doctor's inaccessibility for inseminations*
> *at the right times. At some points, I have gotten so*
> *aggravated that I've considered walking in a bar and*
> *finding my own donor!*

In the midst of focusing on the difficult emotional, legal, and moral issues of donor insemination, it might seem that the negatives outweigh the positives, but that is not so. The many benefits of this procedure should not be forgotten. First, AID is usually successful within six months, compared to the lengthy process of adoption. Success like that is of critical importance after months or years of frustration. Second, the wife will be able to make a genetic contribution to the child, and as one man said, "I'd rather have the baby be half of us than none at all." Finally, the factors surrounding pregnancy and delivery can all be monitored carefully by the couple with their full mutual involvement. There is also the opportunity for the couple to engage in natural childbirth. Many AID couples find this to be particularly satisfying because it provides the husband with an opportunity for involvement, despite the fact that he has not participated biologically. Breast-feeding, too, later becomes an important option.

In conclusion, remember that there are no ironclad answers to any of the questions addressed in this chapter. Each couple must decide on their own answers through honest communication with each other. Regardless of religious background, they must face their personal ethics in contemplating the use of AID. What is right for one person is not necessarily comfortable for another. If the doubts and fears are openly expressed, however, it is far easier to come to terms with this often complicated issue. In the end, AID can be a wonderfully successful means of dealing with infertility and creating the family you have long dreamed about.

In Vitro Fertilization

A *Life* magazine article once referred to in vitro fertilization (IVF) patients as "the most exclusive women's club in America," or probably anywhere else for that matter.[8] Most couples who embark upon this new journey perceive it as a last resort. It is the culmination of countless hours of testing and treatment and the realization that pregnancy, if it is to happen, will come only from the amazing advances of medical technology.

Until 1978, women with absent or damaged fallopian tubes had no hopes of becoming pregnant. Open tubes were essential for conception to occur and medical science had found no form of replacement. Then came the birth of Louise Brown in England, the first in vitro baby, conceived through the efforts of Patrick Steptoe and Robert Edwards. That same year, the first American IVF program opened in Norfolk, Virginia, under the medical direction of Doctors Howard and Georgeanna Jones. Since that time, approximately 200 in vitro clinics have been established around the world, with over 120 now operating in the United States.[9] It is expected that many more will be opening soon.

What Is IVF?

The process of in vitro fertilization may vary somewhat from clinic to clinic, but the following description provides a general idea of what takes place. First, IVF involves surgical removal of eggs from a woman's ovaries. This occurs following regular blood tests and ultra-sound monitoring that have determined when the eggs have sufficiently ripened, but before release from the ovarian follicles. The eggs are removed through a needle while a woman is under general anesthesia and microscopic examination confirms that the fluid taken from the woman's body holds at least one egg. They are then washed, placed in a culture dish filled with nutrients, and incubated for four to eight hours. The husband's sperm are also placed in a solution and then combined with the ova, with the hope that fertilization will occur during the following twenty-four hours. The resulting organism (referred to as a conceptus), after division into two to eight cells, is returned to the woman's uterus in a procedure without anesthesia. The waiting then begins until tests can confirm a pregnancy.

Even the most successful clinics are reporting only 20 percent success rates for pregnancy and most are considerably lower. A worldwide assessment of fifty-eight in vitro programs revealed a 13 percent pregnancy rate per IVF cycle.[10] Many are now placing multiple embryos back in the women's uterus to increase chances of a viable pregnancy. These clinics normally administer drugs such as clomiphene or Pergonal to their patients in an effort to stimulate the ovaries to develop more than the usual single egg each month. The Norfolk program finds that such drug treatment causes an average of 5.8 eggs to develop each month in a patient, and sometimes as many as 17.[11] If several are fertilized and reimplanted, this can contribute to a higher chance of pregnancy but also to a greater likelihood of multiple births.

Who Can Benefit from IVF?

The most likely candidate for IVF is the woman with missing or damaged fallopian tubes. Many such women have unsuccessfully endured microsurgery to attempt repair. Approximately 40 percent of all female infertility problems involve the fallopian tubes, and it is estimated that 490,000 women might, therefore, be candidates for the in vitro procedure.[12]

It has also become a particularly promising option for men with low sperm counts or low motility since the use of this technique places the sperm in close proximity with the egg, thereby eliminating the journey sperm must take through the woman's reproductive tract. Originally, IVF involved only the wife's egg and husband's sperm, but new advances are rapidly being made with other options now available, for example, the use of donor sperm to fertilize the wife's egg. In vitro fertilization is also being used in some cases of unexplained infertility.

Preparing for IVF

Despite enormous media attention to the successes of IVF, there has been little consideration of its tremendous emotional effects and of the fact that success rates at most clinics are not very high. As the number of in vitro centers in the United States is rapidly increasing, it has become crucial to select carefully, for there is great variation in experience and expertise. You need to learn how long a clinic has been in operation, the number of couples who have participated in the program, and their degree of success (number of pregnancies and live births). A word of caution needs to be given regarding success rates, however, since these statistics can be misleading. You need to ask who is included in the statistics (everyone who is accepted in the program or only those from whom mature eggs are harvested) and whether the pregnancy rate includes *clinical* (confirmed by ultrasound) or *chemical* (those that result in very early spontanous abortion) pregnancies. It is generally believed that the inclusion of "chemical pregnancies" in IVF statistics is both misleading and improper. Pregnancy rates can also be presented according to percentage by cycle, by transfer, or by patient. The Norfolk program, for example, from 1981 to 1983 had a pregnancy rate of 18.8 percent by cycle, 24.5 percent by transfer, and 33 percent by patient.[13] Furthermore, pregnancy does not necessarily imply a live birth.

It is also essential that your infertility problems be accurately diagnosed *before* you apply to an in vitro program. Since the better-known programs tend to have long waiting lists, it can be a terrible disappointment to submit your application, wait for months with eager anticipation, and then learn after an evaluation that you are not an appropriate candidate. If considering several programs, try to visit them and assess how comfortable you are with the staff and the environment. It is crucial that you have a sense of confidence and trust in whatever program you choose. For a list of IVF clinics world-wide, write to the American Fertility Society, 2131 Magnolia Avenue, Birmingham, AL 35256.

It is also important that you carefully evaluate your reasons for pursuing the in vitro procedure and are at ease with the decision. Proceeding because your doctor feels it is a good idea and you do not want to disappoint him or her is not a good reason. The same goes for those who feel that they would be "quitters" if they do not force themselves through another endurance test. In vitro fertilization is a *very* involved procedure and requires the full commitment of both partners.

Another part of the preparation for IVF is the anticipation of possible failure. Are you emotionally prepared for it not to work—including the possibilities of no eggs being harvested, fertilization not occurring, a pregnancy test being negative, or your miscarrying? These are all real considerations. Even in the event of success, are you prepared for the possibility of multiple births? Although no one can be totally ready to face these disappointments or surprises, they at least must be seriously weighed beforehand.

The actual experience of in vitro was horrendous for us. The shots and sonograms were painful and scary. My anxiety level was higher than I ever remember and the waiting from one step to the next was almost incapacitating. The fact that the procedure was unsuccessful was, of course, depressing, and the left-over medical bills were ridiculous. The worst thing about having in vitro fail was that my husband and I always felt that if all else failed, we could always do that and end up pregnant. Even though we knew the percentages

*of success, we thought we had better chances (based on
what two doctors told us). So when it didn't work, the
disappointment was extreme. We felt we had nowhere to
go, nothing else to try except in vitro again, which
would be a nightmare relived. It's taken a couple of
months to recover from the in vitro experience, and we
are just now actively involving ourselves again in
infertility matters.*

The Experience of IVF

The IVF procedure is an all-consuming one, and once you are en-
gulfed in it, it may be difficult to focus on anything but the daily
procedures of blood tests, sonograms, and hormone injections. It
bombards your body physically and emotionally. At a place like the
Norfolk clinic, emotions run so high that patients experience an
immediate bonding with one another and a family atmosphere often
develops. Infertility histories are quickly and openly shared with
constant discussion of drugs, blocked tubes, and ectopic pregnancies, not to mention the hopes and fears. In many, if not most, of the
programs, though, little is offered in the way of professional emotional help from the clinical staff. This makes it extremely important
to have the support of family, friends, or new relationships with
other infertile couples at the facility.

*There were months of preparation for IVF—blood tests,
sperm tests, a psychological evaluation, making
arrangements for time off from work, and making
plans to stay with relatives. That was just for starters.
When the procedure actually began, I spent eight days
traveling back and forth to the hospital twice a
day—at 7:30 A.M. for blood work, pelvic exams, and
sonograms, and then back at 4:00 for my Pergonal shot.
Even though this was very tiring emotionally, it was a
"high." Everyday you would be getting closer to
achieving that long-awaited dream—a pregnancy.
Talking and sharing feelings with the other women
going through the program was a great help. We were
like a family, each of us rooting for the other person. I
wanted all of us to become pregnant. You couldn't help*

but feel optimistic, but you had to face the fact that it might not work. You had to be prepared for the worst or the best. I guess that's why it's such a stressful, emotional experience.

Owing to a death in the family, we had to stop before egg removal, but the doctors encouraged us to try it naturally. For about two weeks after returning home, I became very depressed—more so than I've ever been. I cried a lot and felt very hopeless about ever having a child. In fact, I didn't want anything to do with pursuing pregnancy. Sleep was the only thing I wanted to do. Thanks to my husband, friends, and family, I slowly began feeling better. Eventually, I bounced back and my hope returned. I began thinking about future in vitro procedures and the possibility of adoption. I learned from this experience, though, just how powerful emotions can be. Despite all this, I will try in vitro fertilization again, just because there is hope for a possible child through this method.

IVF was the next and only remaining step for us to take, so there was no question but to try it. We are still working on it. The overall experience has been good—the team is supportive, the program is interesting, and it is our hope. However, on a day-to-day, month-to-month basis, it feels like a roller coaster—stressful, exhausting, draining. Some days you are very positive and hopeful, while others are full of despair and discouragement. Generally, though, it is a good experience and allows me to postpone casting a final verdict of "infertile" upon myself.

Attempts at IVF often become addictive. Hope and desperation are so intense that there is always the fantasy that "next time" will be "it," encouraging couples to keep on trying. Some programs will allow you to continue efforts for as long as desired, whereas others limit the attempts or require a certain number of months between trials. Waiting until the next opportunity can be frustrating. Each try can bring a somewhat better chance, in that the clinic becomes more knowledgeable about a particular patient. But the emotional and financial toll are enormous. Each monthly procedure in the United States, excluding travel expenses, hotel bills, and lost salary, amounts to $3,000 to $5,000, with insurance coverage presently very limited.

Anxiety does not dissipate even with the confirmation that pregnancy has occurred. Unfortunately, a third of the women who conceive will have miscarriages in the first trimester. Many with normally progressing pregnancies also worry about the possibility of an abnormal baby, probably owing in large part to the unusual means of conception. To allay such fears, it should be remembered that all of the IVF children thus far delivered have been healthy and normal, except for one baby with a nongenetic heart defect.

Delivering a baby conceived through IVF, on the other hand, has been described as a thrill beyond imagination. At this point, there appear to be no regrets or misgivings about the manner of conception. Intensely positive feelings toward the physician and other medical staff involved are also common.

How Society Views IVF

Some couples are plagued by worries about how their neighbors will perceive them. Unfortunately, in contrast to the hopeful anticipation and excitement of the IVF process, it may be shocking for many couples if they are criticized or questioned about their efforts. Because of the explosion of publicity over Louise Brown's birth in England and the later proliferation of IVF centers in the United States, it is a topic that everyone knows about and has an opinion on. As with most aspects of infertility, though, the public also tends to have misconceptions about the in vitro process. This may, in part, be due to the term *test-tube baby*, which feeds fantasies of babies developing in glass containers. Most people involved with infertility find this expression to be not only inaccurate but distasteful. As more realistic information becomes available and the sensational publicity declines, the public should develop a more accurate understanding of the procedure.

Two polls taken in 1978 found that the majority of people questioned were in favor of IVF being offered as a choice for an infertile couple.[14] Those opposed to it have voiced their views loudly, however, and have given numerous reasons for their stance. Some feel that physicians are taking God's will into their own hands.

Others state that medical intervention has intruded upon a natural, loving event and transformed it into a mechanical, artificial process that destroys the meaning of family. Perhaps the most significant of the protests, however, involves the fear that IVF represents only a beginning step in what could become the manipulation of human life through altering conception. Some fear, for example, that technology will reach the point where couples could decide what traits they want in their children by selecting among eggs in a "bank" or that researchers might eventually try to cross-breed other species with human beings.

Legal Concerns about IVF

All this illustrates just how perplexing and worrisome the legal and ethical questions about IVF can be. Although more and more babies conceived through IVF are being born in the United States, no specific legal provisions have been made for these offspring. What laws do exist pertain only to the procedure itself. Following the legalization of abortion in 1973, many states have passed laws regarding restrictions on "experimentation" with fetuses. The question of rights concerning the embryo that is sitting in a petri dish is mind-boggling. For example, if more than one embryo develops during the IVF process, must all of them be reimplanted and in whom—the mother or other infertile women? If not reimplanted, should they be destroyed, frozen, or used in other research?

The issues could become politically explosive; so many are not anxious to touch them. Walter Wadlington, a University of Virginia law professor quoted in the *Wall Street Journal*, said, "There is a great danger in doing nothing. We are not going to get very far by having things come to the courts piecemeal. But the problems have been ignored so long that when the legislatures do try to act, they will have so many competing interests to deal with."[15] Some states that seem to be ignoring the issue are, perhaps, overwhelmed by the speed with which the new technologies are progressing.

The first state to address the use of IVF was Illinois in 1979. Strangely, the courts there stated that any physician engaging in IVF would become "legal custodian of the embryo and liable for possible prosecution under an 1877 law against child abuse."[16] This obviously put Illinois doctors in a precarious position, and although the law did not actually ban use of IVF, it has made many physicians reluctant to take the risk. Since it is presently state law that rules on family issues, doctor-patient relationships, and embryo experimentation, it is essential that you become aware of the positions of your own state or of the state in which a clinic is located.

Final Considerations

Anyone enduring the throes of infertility will recognize the value of the IVF procedure and the joy such a "miracle" can bring to couples otherwise unable to bear children. If you are considering in vitro fertilization, however, do enter this process in a realistic manner. First, keep in mind that it is a relatively new procedure, and therefore, further study is needed to refine it and investigate the unknowns. Second, the rate for successful pregnancies is still low, except in the most experienced programs (although progress is occurring). And finally, IVF is costly in time, effort, money, and emotions. It is worth everything if a baby results, but you must face the situation with your mind clear and your eyes wide open. Know the facts—don't rush in expecting miracles.

Surrogate Parenting

If you witness the joy and excitement of an infertile couple who have just had a child through surrogate parenting, the procedure would seem to be a wonderful solution to the problem of infertility. And for them, it has been. Yet the use of surrogates is condemned by many and perceived as the most controversial of the new conceptions.

What Is Surrogate Parenting?

Surrogate parenting is increasingly used as an option in situations where the husband is fertile, but the wife cannot or should not get pregnant owing to a variety of infertility problems or pregnancy risks.

The procedure involves the artificial insemination of a donor, or surrogate female, with sperm from the husband. This woman carries the baby to term and, following delivery, relinquishes the child to the couple. Since the husband is the biological father, only the wife must legally adopt the baby. From a medical standpoint the process is simple, but it involves complex ethical considerations. Many think that surrogate parenting is immoral because a woman is intentionally creating a life with the sole purpose of handing it over to another for a price. The arrangement to them smacks of "baby-selling." Others are apprehensive about the technique because the lengthy commitment and deep involvement of the surrogate make it a rich ground for serious conflict.

Although surrogate parenting is a new option in modern society, it may surprise you to know that it was practiced in ancient cultures. Even the Bible (Genesis 16:1–2) refers to the use of surrogating when wives were found to be barren.

The procedure today has been in use since the late 1970s, and well over 150 children have been conceived under such agreements.[17] Noel Keane, a Michigan attorney, pioneered the concept in 1976 and has become an expert on the many legal questions it has created. He developed a program in Dearborn, Michigan, and, more recently, one in New York City (the Infertility Center of New York). A variety of other centers have also opened throughout the United States, some of which include Surrogate Mothering, Ltd. (Philadelphia), The Association for Surrogate Parenting Services (Corona Del Mar, California), Hagar Institute (Topeka, Kansas), Surrogate Parenting Associates, Inc. (Louisville, Kentucky), and Sherwyn and Handel (Beverly Hills). These centers and others vary greatly in the selection of surrogates, the amount and nature of contacts with the surrogate mother, the legal provisions, and the costs (which can amount to over $30,000). Some couples also advertise or make other private arrangements to obtain a surrogate.

The Advantages of Using a Surrogate Mother

Why does a couple choose surrogate parenting? Many point out the positive aspects of this option in contrast to adoption. Couples feel that, as in donor insemination, they are at least contributing half of the genetic material to their baby. And they like being able to select carefully the woman who will be the mother. The couple receives information regarding her health, educational background, level of intelligence, motivation, emotional stability, and physical characteristics. In some programs, they have the opportunity to meet her. By following the pregnancy, they maintain some sense of control through their knowledge of the situation. Compared to adoption, then, there are fewer unknowns.

Many, too, feel that from the beginning the baby is conceived "for them," again in contrast to adoption. It is also believed that a surrogate experiences less emotional conflict about her role than does a woman with an unforeseen or unwanted pregnancy, and that the baby is not being "given up" or "abandoned."

Another major difference between surrogate parenting and adoption is that the latter, especially when pursued through agencies, will usually take far longer to complete. Surrogate parenting may be an especially good option for women in their late or even postchildbearing years, since adoption agencies often deny the applications of couples past their late thirties. Knowing that the surrogate option exists also allows a couple whatever time is necessary to attempt other treatments. For example, if a woman at age thirty-seven suddenly learns that she has tubal blockage, the availability of surrogate parenting can alleviate her panic; she can turn to that option if efforts to overcome her medical problem fail. The new option, then, brings hope to couples who otherwise may have reached the end of the road.

Finally, there is the appealing feature of its success rate. Compared to other alternatives that also require large financial and emotional investments, surrogate parenting has a high degree of success.

The Emotional Impact of Surrogate Parenting

Surrogate parenting, although simple in technique, is emotionally a very complicated experience. The similarities between the feelings of a man considering AID and a woman weighing the issues of surrogating are apparent, but additional problems exist for her. First, AID is used in secrecy and the pregnancy that results is treated by the rest of the world as "normal." Moreover, the wife is carrying the baby, and the couple can easily relate to it as "their own." This is different from the experience of surrogate parenting, regardless of how much contact they have with the surrogate. They must experience the pregnancy vicariously, and social supports may be nonexistent. In addition, it will probably be the wife who will spend the bulk of her time with the child, and yet, from a medical standpoint, she is the person least involved in the procedure.

It is crucial that the wife first resolve her feelings about her infertility and then confront her reactions to the idea of a surrogate. Will she feel that the child is "their baby" or just her husband's? Will she resent the surrogate mother's ability to bear a child and the woman's genetic contribution? Will she feel excluded from the process? Does she fear that the child will lack a loving bond to her? She must be reasonably certain of her feelings toward the other woman and the procedure *before* embarking on the project. Even so, there is apt to be an initial sense of despondency in pursuing surrogate parenting when the wife feels that she is not included in the procedure.

Couples should understand that several attempts at insemination (often taking four to six months) may be necessary before pregnancy results, and sometimes all efforts may be unsuccessful. In the latter situation, they may need to choose another surrogate. Obviously, this can be frustrating and anxiety provoking for all concerned. While waiting for conception to occur, couples and surrogates may have second thoughts about their decision to enter the arrangement. Support from family and friends can be crucial at this time to endure the anxiety.

Once pregnancy occurs and the couple can begin to share the excitement of a developing baby, any early doubts and despondency will probably vanish, although anxiety will still flourish. The wife may feel jealous of the surrogate, too, which she should acknowledge and work through.

A few words of caution: (1) a wife who is uncomfortable with the idea but agrees to surrogate parenting because her husband is opposed to adoption or insists on his own genetic input is setting herself up for future problems; (2) using this procedure to cement a failing marriage without resolving feelings about one's infertility and the option itself is also a surefire way to create difficulties, not solve them; and (3) a couple who searches endlessly for the "perfect" surrogate with unique traits may be indicating that they have not resolved their feelings about the procedure. Although selection should take place carefully, it is essential that both partners understand their motivations in pursuing this option.

Selecting a Surrogate

Once you have decided that surrogate parenting is a comfortable choice, a variety of concerns regarding selection of the surrogate is likely to surface.

1. Is it better to choose a surrogate who is previously unknown to you or to work with a close friend or relative who has offered her help?

Some couples have chosen a family member or friend to act as the surrogate because they find the situation comforting, at least initially. It also may save on expenses. This decision can create a problem later, however, for it may open a Pandora's box of feelings and issues. Here are some important questions to consider:

A. How will you eventually perceive the relationship and special union between your husband and the close friend or relative who has served as surrogate?

B. Since contact between the child and surrogate is likely to continue throughout the years to come, how will you react to their relationship? Will you feel threatened by their biological bond?

C. What, if anything, have you planned to tell your child about the conception? If you choose to keep the circumstances secret or to tell the child that he was adopted, how will you handle the fact that family and friends are aware of the surrogate arrangement?

It is not impossible to use a surrogate with whom you are closely associated, but everyone involved must thoroughly examine the issues beforehand.

If you decide to use a surrogate parenting center, the selection of surrogates will vary according to the center you select. At the Infertility Center of New York, applicants for becoming a surrogate mother must complete a questionnaire regarding medical history, personal data (age, height, weight, color of hair and eyes), educational background, and motivations for applying. Couples interested in finding a surrogate examine a file of these applications, including pictures, in search of a woman with whom they feel most comfortable or who seems to best suit their needs. In contrast, other centers, after extensive interviewing, make the selection for the couple. This choice, of course, is subject to the couple's approval.

In contacting a center, feel free to ask plenty of questions: How are surrogates screened, medically and emotionally? What are the legal responsibilities and rights of all involved? What kind and amount of contact is there between the couple and the surrogate? Is counseling provided for surrogates and couples? Many of the centers operate with a group of professionals (physicians, attorneys, psychologists, and other mental health workers), and it is important that you ask to meet all these people since they, together, will be contributing to the experience. Centers offering surrogate parenting services are required by the American College of Obstetrics and Gynecology to evaluate both the surrogate mothers and the couples from a psychological and medical standpoint. As in any service, however, but especially one where standards are vague, some will handle this more thoroughly and professionally than others.

Since the procedure can be stressful for both couples and surrogates, it is crucial that counseling be available. Some centers, in fact, require that all surrogates participate in counseling sessions. No matter how prepared the couple and surrogate feel they are, problems are bound to come up. As one surrogate related, "[At the end] you don't feel the same way you did at the beginning. . . . I didn't think it would bother me at all. But it did. I was totally naive when I first started. It was very, very hard."[18]

Surrogates, too, may have their own ideas in deciding to contract with a particular couple. There are many reasons for women pursuing the opportunity to be surrogate mothers, besides a need for money. Some have a history of easy pregnancies and enjoy the special feelings of the experience. Others may need to dispel guilt over a previous abortion or may feel an altruistic desire to help infertile couples because of personal contact with the hardships of infertility through a friend or relative. A few may simply feel that it is an important cause and want to make a positive contribution to society. As one surrogate stated, "People donate things—kidneys, livers, eyes—after they're gone. This is something you can donate when you're alive."[19]

2. How much and what kind of contact with the surrogate is beneficial?

Whether a couple wishes to have direct contact with their surrogate needs to be carefully considered. Contact during the pregnancy may be enjoyable or even thrilling, in that the experience of carrying the baby is shared and a strong feeling of involvement is created. It also may foster, for the surrogate, an even clearer sense of what she is accomplishing for this couple. In fact, some feel that the development of the couple-surrogate relationship may further decrease the risk of the surrogate changing her mind because she may feel stronger loyalty toward the people with whom she has contracted. On the other hand, and perhaps more important, the postpregnancy time must be taken into consideration. Having developed a relationship with the surrogate, how might you feel after the baby is born? Will this relationship intrude upon your own bonding with the baby? Many couples worry that a surrogate might later try to interfere in raising the child.

At some centers, very close relationships develop between the couple, particularly the wife, and the surrogate. The wife may even serve as the labor coach, with both husband and wife present at the delivery. The relationship between the wife and the surrogate becomes more than just "womanly" sharing—it can be an intensely vicarious experience for the wife who is unable to carry a baby, a way of strongly involving herself in a process from which she is medically absent, and perhaps a way of mastering any jealous feelings over the "relationship" between her husband and the surrogate. The surrogate, in such situations, often forms an equally dependent feeling toward the couple. As noted earlier, though, you must consider how to handle this closeness once the baby is born.

Surrogate parenting centers may feel strongly about their own approach to the question of contact (which vary from no contact whatever to ongoing face-to-face visits), so you must clarify this issue from the outset. There is a middle-of-the-road position that may be comfortable for you—meeting with the surrogate on one occasion before signing the contract and then having ongoing communication during the pregnancy through a third person (physician, attorney) or through correspondence. Many feel this arrangement provides a sense of emotional closeness and sharing, but also some degree of distance. If you do decide to have contact (physical or written) with your surrogate, it is important to be aware of her feelings in this procedure. Surrogates often state that they want the couple to be considerate of their physical and emotional well-being during the pregnancy, not just being treated as a "baby-making machine."

3. How can you be assured of the baby's care in utero? Will the surrogate refrain from drinking alcohol, smoking, and taking drugs? Will she eat properly?

There is no way to guarantee that a surrogate is handling the pregnancy correctly, but maintaining regular contact with her or getting information through a third-party professional can be helpful. This may assure you that the pregnancy is proceeding smoothly and that the surrogate is taking good care of herself and the baby during these months.

4. Will the surrogate honor the contract and not claim the baby for herself?

No matter how comfortable and confident you feel with the surrogate, there is probably always some degree of apprehension regarding her ultimate decision to release the baby to your care, and unfortunately, there can be no absolute assurance that she will uphold the agreement. Under present law, this aspect of the contract is not binding, although a couple could initiate legal proceedings should the surrogate refuse to relinquish the baby.

Here are some questions you may want to ask in order to decrease the chances of this happening:

A. What is the surrogate trying to get out of the experience? You need to explore her motivation and evaluate how sincere she appears in expressing her reasons for becoming a surrogate.

B. How stable is her personal life and does she have a support system? The more stable her life is and the more supports she has, the greater the likelihood of the contract being upheld.

C. What is the attitude of the surrogate's husband? You certainly do not want him to oppose the contract and apply pressure on his wife to change her mind.

D. How reliable does the surrogate appear to be? Is there anything in her history to suggest erratic or irresponsible behavior? It is difficult to predict the future, but a woman with a fairly stable history and a responsible character offers a better gamble.

E. Does the surrogate have children of her own? Some professionals involved with surrogate parenting feel that there are advantages when the surrogate has previously had children. Not only does it ensure that she is aware of what is in store for her regarding the pregnancy and delivery, but it may also make it easier for her to release the baby for adoption if she has a family of her own.

These factors may not guarantee a successful ending, but they offer at least some guidelines. Maintaining some contact with the surrogate along the way may diminish your normal worries.

How to Explain the Decision to Others

Another important aspect of the surrogate parenting process, from an emotional point of view, involves who the couple plan to tell, what they plan to tell, and when. Of all the infertility options, this one may incite the greatest opposition from others who fail to understand the motivation for using a surrogate.

The issues of who, what, and when may depend a great deal on what you eventually plan to explain to your child about the conception. Many centers, including the Hagar Institute in Kansas, recommend that parents be honest with their child from the beginning, encouraging open discussion. Some couples, however, have decided simply to tell others that a child has been adopted, without going into details. They also plan to keep the surrogate procedure secret from the child. This obviously is a personal decision to be made by you and your spouse. I can offer no rule of thumb, and, to my knowledge, no research has been done on the issue. If you do decide to tell others about using a surrogate, remember that it may take time for them to understand and become adjusted to the idea.

Legal Implications of Surrogate Parenting

From a legal standpoint, surrogate parenting is a complex and risky practice, and those who engage in it need to be aware of the pitfalls. Here are a few of the legal questions that can arise:

1. What happens if the baby is born handicapped or seriously ill?

2. Is the contract changed in any way should something happen to the husband prior to the baby's birth?

3. If the surrogate breaks the contract, can the couple be reimbursed?

4. What rights does the husband have if the surrogate refuses to relinquish the child for adoption?

5. What happens if the couple's relationship deteriorates and they decide to separate or divorce during the pregnancy?

This is uncharted territory. No state yet has established provisions guiding the procedure, although twenty-four carry statutes on the subject of adoption that, in general, prohibit any monies from being paid to a woman who gives up her child. State legislation regarding AID and family issues may also have some bearing on surrogate parenting. For example, in many states, family law mandates that the husband of any woman who gets pregnant during the marriage is presumed to be the father of the child, and the courts often will not even admit blood tests or other evidence to show that he could not actually have fathered the child.[20] A number of states are in the process of specifying legal guidelines, but these legislative bills vary greatly. Some propose freedom to practice surrogating, whereas others plan to make it illegal.

Legislation is undoubtedly needed to monitor the procedure to protect the well-being of all concerned and to lessen the risks involved. In the meantime, you should examine the laws in your own state before making any arrangements. The sensationalistic manner in which surrogate parenting has been handled has created some drawbacks, and the high financial cost of surrogate centers puts this option out of reach for many couples. Others may be cynical about the arrangement and regard it as a money-making venture for both the centers and the surrogates. But if you are an infertile couple and this is your last resort, you will see it from a different perspective— it is the opportunity to hold a baby in your arms that you have helped create and that is yours to love. In the end, the option will be comfortable for some, but not for others. Still, it should be a choice.

The Crossroads
of Infertility

In a way, learning to live with infertility is like
learning to live with death; one can't quite forget about
it, but one can't think about it all the time.[1]

Chances are you have traveled from one infertility test and treatment to the next, always hoping for success. But now time has passed and frustrations have grown, and you are facing last resorts. You have hit the crossroads of infertility.

Arriving at the crossroads means that you are about to accept the reality of infertility, that you are beginning to come to terms with its impact on your life. The ultimate decisions must be made: Do you still want children? How are you going to accomplish this? No matter how painful, the questions must be answered.

For some, this point will come abruptly, as in the case of a woman who has had unsuccessful tubal surgery and is confronted with her inability to conceive. For others, the need for final decision making will evolve in a slow, gradual manner, as in the case of a couple with unexplained infertility who have searched fruitlessly for answers.

Finding the strength to make these decisions and to resolve feelings about infertility will, for most of you, be triggered by an event. Your sister may make one last, hurtful comment and your crying has left you drained; your doctor suggests still another treatment and you find that you don't have the energy or the will to try it; or you've been offered a job promotion, and for one last time, you're torn by the conflict of treatment schedules versus career demands. Sometimes the event is some dramatic blow, but more than likely it's just the straw that breaks the camel's back. It catalyzes a final episode of grieving, which in turn helps push you toward resolution. Experiences like these suddenly make you realize that enough is enough. It's time to move on.

The Meaning of Resolution

Many think that finally delivering a baby, or adopting one, signifies resolution, but this is not so. The memories and experiences of infertility, and the changes these have wrought, are not whisked away by a baby's cry. Resolution is achieved emotionally, not physically. It is an endpoint that occurs only after considerable time—time to accept that infertility has been a reality in your life, time to respond to the fear and pain it has inflicted upon you, and time to gather strength to weather the crisis. Resolution means that you have finally put into perspective all those months or years of trying to have a baby.

Infertility has become a popular subject in recent years, with an abundance of articles, books, and talk shows dealing with it. Unfortunately, the hype and the media coverage has been a mixed blessing. The attention helps make the public more aware of the problems facing infertile couples, but it also presents a distorted picture. In the media, infertility ends happily in only one way—a beautiful, bouncing baby is biologically produced by the infertile couple. This is the fairy-tale ending whereby everyone lives happily ever after. It sounds terrific, but it's not very realistic. First, many infertile couples do not experience this ending, and yet their outcome is not sad or uncomfortable—just different. Second, the media, while extolling happy endings, avoid the suffering that infertility has caused and the scars that remain. The years of struggle are never instantly erased. In fact, the emotional effects may never disappear completely, especially for those who cannot fulfill their dream of having biological children. As one woman said at the end of her long struggle with infertility:

> *I do know . . . from other wounds, that healing means only that—it is healed; that it is healed does not mean it never happened. The scar is always there; the broken place is vulnerable and may ache on bad days. I know what it was like before; I'm different now; and I will never be the same.*[2]

To neglect this fact is to fail to understand what infertility really is, what it does to people, and why it is so difficult to resolve.

Achieving resolution means several things: making sense out of confusion; building bridges where relationships have been severed; accepting a future that is perhaps different than expected; and, most important, making peace with yourself. It means that intense feelings have been overcome and you can look ahead with optimism. It is the knowledge that there really can be life after infertility.

Approaching Resolution

Considerably more is asked of the infertile couple than of those who are fertile. They must answer many difficult questions, all a part of resolving the crisis. For example:

> What are your motivations for becoming parents?
>
> How important is the experience of pregnancy to you?
>
> How do you feel about alternative means of conception?
>
> Would adoption be comfortable, and if so, what are your specific needs?
>
> Could you adopt and raise a baby from another country?
>
> Is an older, special needs child a responsibility you could handle?
>
> Would it be better to try AID than to adopt?

These are just a few of the issues that require soul-searching. Fertile individuals have probably never had to face the prejudices tucked inside that you must openly admit and confront. Issues of heredity, race, and ethnicity all must be tackled.

Another important question involves your beliefs regarding environment versus heredity. For example, if you believe that a child is a product only of genetics and that environment has little influence, it might be very difficult for you to adopt a child. How many fertile couples struggle with this issue before becoming parents?

Despite the fact that families are diverse in today's society (50 percent of all families in the United States today are not biological in origin), most people still retain the traditional notion of the normal family—Mom, Dad, and two or more biologically produced children. Considering having a different type of family, whether through adoption or medical technology, can be difficult, as typified by this couple's struggle:

> *We approached adoption with great hesitancy, but had the great fortune to come upon a very nice and capable adoption worker. She listened to all our concerns about adoption and then said, "Well, why are you here since you don't like the idea of adoption?" I replied, "You've listened to our garbage; maybe now I'll think of some good things about adoption."*

When to Stop Trying

One of the reasons resolution of infertility is such a struggle lies within the field itself. Diagnoses are often complex, uncertain, or even nonexistent. And treatments are diverse, often experimental. To complicate matters, infertility is a condition in which the patient often has a strong hand in the treatment, guiding it and setting the pace. Although this is a positive aspect, it presents a dilemma when it comes to resolution. There is no doctor saying, "You must stop. There's no point in continuing." Because absolute accuracy is rarely possible in this specialty, doctors are reluctant to recommend an end. That means that only you, the couple, can make that very difficult decision.

> *Only time has helped us to finally reach resolution. I needed to try and try again, and give a lot of time and energy into conceiving first. I also had to accept the idea of adoption—that's taken over a year. That decision (which isn't finished yet) has been very difficult. I feel at times like I'm letting society down, my family down, myself down, and my husband down. Sometimes I feel I should hang in there. Now, though, I feel that it is okay to hang it up and move on, but I still feel a twinge of guilt—that I owe it to the world or someone to keep going through these ridiculous tests to prove that I'm a fighter.*

How do you know when it's time to quit the medical heroics?

Unfortunately, there are no clear-cut answers, but addressing the following questions should help you assess your present position and make your decision:

1. Have you exhausted all the medical possibilities that you feel comfortable pursuing?

2. Are you feeling that the role of parent is more important to you than pregnancy?

3. Do you hate the fact that infertility has taken over your life to the extent that little else matters?

4. Do your present efforts at treatment seem hopeless?

5. Are you now able to discuss alternative means of parenthood that, in the past, were off limits?

6. Do you dream of resuming a normal life again with laughter and happiness as a couple?

7. Do you hate the kind of person you've become—dull, depressed, and irritable?

8. Do you feel angry and resentful on days when you are scheduled to see your doctor?

9. Does an end to temperature taking, drugs, and doctors' appointments sound like a relief?

10. Would you feel unhappy if your doctor informed you that a wonderful new treatment had just become available?

11. Are you just plain tired?

If you find yourself answering yes to the majority of these questions, chances are you are ready to consider alternative means of conception like AID or an end to treatment altogether with adoption or childfree living as your new goal. In some cases, couples find that they are able to begin efforts to adopt and continue medical treatment at the same time. This dual effort is often a comfortable stepping stone in the direction of adoption and does not necessarily indicate conflicted feelings about pursuing that route. Many feel a sense of relief when they initiate adoption inquiries, but they still want to keep the dream of biological parenthood alive.

If your positive responses to the question above are in the minority, it would indicate that your motivation and spirits are still relatively high and that there is value in continuing your efforts toward biological parenthood. Reassess your answers to these questions periodically, however, to be aware when the need for resolution is approaching.

The point at which resolution occurs comes at different times for different people and may be precipitated by a variety of events. The following are two such experiences:

> *It took a long time, but I was finally able to look at myself and admit that I didn't like what I'd become or what my life had turned into. I was miserable and my life was going nowhere. I was obsessed with getting pregnant and could barely think of anything else. The news of another's pregnancy would send me into a funk for days. But then it happened—a tremendous low which was the culmination of unsuccessful surgery and three close friends getting pregnant all at once. I suddenly realized that I had had it and I needed to get a grip on myself. Resolution was only starting for me then, but that's all I needed—a start.*

> *One day I was traveling into the city for a full schedule of doctors' appointments. I was exhausted and terribly anxious about what my sonogram would show that day. It was ridiculously hot, the traffic was unbearable, and I was worried that I'd never get back to work on time. For a moment, I thought I might actually snap from all the pressure. Then suddenly I realized that I just couldn't go through this anymore. It had become too much. Believe it or not, I made a U-turn at the next exit and came home. That was my last scheduled appointment.*

Ending infertility treatment, then, can be a sudden decision or a gradually realized step, especially with new medical opportunities cropping up regularly. But sometime there has to be an end. It helps if you and your spouse can work together to develop a realistic timetable. And along the way, make sure you know how your partner feels about stopping.

Getting Stuck

There are so many pieces of the infertility process to handle before arriving at resolution that many couples get stuck along the way, spinning their wheels in a fruitless effort to have a baby and digging themselves deeper and deeper into depression and misery. Some may not even realize how stuck they are. When you are obsessed with your goal and consumed by anger, denial, or guilt, it is hard to be rational in assessing your position.

The following signs might indicate that you are at a serious standstill:

1. You or your spouse refuse to admit that an infertility problem even exists, despite prolonged efforts to conceive, or you refuse to believe a physician who says there is a medical problem requiring treatment. When denial of this nature is long-lasting and steadfastly maintained, a critical situation exists. You are not facing reality.

2. Physicians are pessimistic, indicating there is little, if any, chance of a successful pregnancy, but you continue to try (even after second and third opinions from specialists).

3. You've been trying for so long and become so obsessed that your life has lost all joy and other purpose.

4. Efforts to conceive have long been unsuccessful and yet you refuse to even consider alternative measures, such as AID, in vitro fertilization, or adoption.

Experiencing any one of these situations may indicate that you are stuck. It is extremely important that you begin to reassess your infertility predicament or seek help in understanding what is happening.

Sometimes people are unable to get beyond their rage about infertility, refusing to acknowledge or accept that this is a situation over which they have little control. This can be a common problem for success-oriented individuals who cannot believe they are not always masters of their fate. They depend on a high level of achievement to give them a positive sense of themselves. Inability to produce a child makes them see themselves as imperfect, which goes against their grain. They may project their anger onto their spouse or the professionals involved in their treatment, in some cases, never admitting the anger to themselves. If they do not recognize its existence, they cannot work it through.

For others, unsuccessful resolution is the result of guilt. These people often see themselves as terrible persons who deserve their infertility. They may develop masochistic behavior as a means of atoning for their sins. Barbara Eck Menning notes how frequently such people will suddenly decide to take on work with unwed mothers, maternity patients, or abortion counseling as a masochistic way of purging themselves.[3]

Inability to grieve can also lead to getting stuck. Some may be unable to talk about their infertility, feeling it is too personal, shameful, or embarrassing. Others may be afraid that if they allow their grief to surface, they will be overwhelmed or devastated in a flood of emotion. The consoling fact is that grieving is really time limited; it will be painful, but it ends. Some may feel uncertain about their infertility, especially if a diagnosis is not clear-cut. They do not want to mourn until they are sure there is something to mourn about. Menning compares this situation to the difficulty of grieving when a soldier is missing in action—you are never sure. Finally, there are those who find the loss intangible and, therefore, do not perceive infertility as a true source of bereavement. The situation does not represent for them a death as such, except perhaps in the case of miscarriage. Instead, it is the end of a dream and the loss of an ability, rather than a child.

If inability to grieve is at the core of your difficulty in moving on, you may have to push yourself to start feeling. Rather than fighting off the emotion, you must let yourself feel its impact. Begin to picture what the biological child you've longed for would look like: Would it be a boy or a girl? What color hair and eyes would it have? Who would the baby look like? Imagine yourself holding the baby close to you and rocking back and forth. Force yourself to walk into baby stores and look at the tiny clothing and shoes. Imagine yourself and your spouse sharing the joy of a baby with family and friends. Think about how old the child would be now if you hadn't been infertile. Would you be playing ball in the backyard or taking trips to the zoo? For some people, these fantasies are close to the surface and will easily prompt periods of grief. Others, whose emotions and dreams have been kept tightly in check, need to face the depth of their feelings and allow themselves to mourn.

The problem of getting stuck may also result from people identifying so strongly with their parents that they cannot tolerate the idea of being different from them, of not having a family as they did. Buried in this feeling may be the fear that their parents will reject them because of their failure.

Professional help is usually necessary when chronic problems develop as a result of not resolving infertility. Although these people may appear only normally sad on the surface, their underlying feelings of guilt or anger may be so intense and unacceptable that they unconsciously block awareness of them and cannot handle them.

Successfully resolving infertility does not mean that the feelings are gone forever, only that they have been acknowledged and worked through.

Each day I look at my son and can hardly believe my eyes that he is really mine. I still feel very much infertile, and I don't think that I'll ever get over that feeling.

You may have to deal with your feelings regarding infertility again and again throughout your life, but they will subside as the years go on. Most come to accept that the feelings will quietly exist, surfacing only at vulnerable moments.

Understanding Your Needs

Understanding your needs and separating the experience of pregnancy from that of being a parent may clarify how best to end your infertility dilemma. Of course, this is an ongoing issue during infertility; but as you approach resolution it must be reassessed one final time. Originally you may not have been aware of your motivations, or perhaps your feelings have changed.

Most infertile people probably long for both the pregnancy and the parenting experience, although there are some who focus more on one than the other. Try to assess where your desires lie and whether one of these is more important to you. Ask yourself which goal you are pursuing. There is nothing wrong with wanting a pregnancy for the experience of being pregnant, but you need to know if that or parenthood is your primary aim. Because it may sound selfish or narcissistic, you might find it difficult to acknowledge a wish for

*parents. When this is not the case, there is bound to be
disappointment and regret, because a baby is primarily
made up of needs, and it is his needs that must be
gratified by the parent, and not the other way around.
Furthermore, there is no guarantee of eventual return or
reward for providing the needs of a child. Parenthood is
a giving, guiding, full-time responsibility that lasts
forever. Once a parent, always a parent.*[4]

Ideally, people should have children when they feel confidence
and merit in themselves and when they have a relatively good understanding of and appreciation for who they are. Obviously, this
does not always happen, though. Most people enter into parenthood
with relatively little thought as to their motivations and without full
emotional maturity. As miserable as infertility is, it does provide the
time and opportunity to assess yourself and determine what you
need and want.

Assessing Your Motivations

Understanding your personal motivations regarding pregnancy and
parenthood will not only be an asset in your own development, but
also in your role as parent should you choose this responsibility. This
understanding will also help you clarify which means of resolution
will best suit your needs.

*I have always known that I wanted to be a parent, but
infertility has given me time to examine my reasons for
this desire. I still know that I want to have children but
now am more comfortable with my motivation to work
toward that goal.*

*I'm more excited than ever about being a parent. I also
think that we will be better parents because of our
infertility experience. I now know what really matters
in life, and I'm stronger, wiser, more sensitive, and
kinder.*

*I still would love to have the experience of pregnancy
but now realize that it's the role of being a parent that*

I most want. Clarifying that for myself has helped greatly in learning to accept the need for adoption.

It is possible, too, that when you examine your feelings about pregnancy and parenthood you will become aware of inner doubts.

I can't honestly say anymore why I want a child— maybe I never really knew in the first place. At this point, I suspect much of the time it's because I'm pissed off that I couldn't make the choice. I wonder why I've become so obsessed and if it is all worth it.

It is not uncommon for people to battle for years against infertility, assuming that their struggle is to have children, when actually it is a struggle simply to become fertile. No one likes to have a choice taken from them, especially one as important as parenthood. If you find it difficult to imagine a life with children, and the changes that entails, it may be that your fight for fertility has been just that—a fight to have the *choice* to conceive, not necessarily to have children. A book that may be helpful to those of you in this situation is *The Baby Decision* by Merle Bombardieri. She closely examines the issues in choosing whether or not to become a parent and provides guidelines for making the decision.

As you examine your feelings about pregnancy and parenthood, try making a list of all the things you originally looked forward to in both these experiences, and assign priorities to them. Then consider how many you could achieve by the alternatives you are now contemplating. Putting it down in black and white may clarify your position.

Remember that there are three outcomes to infertility: (1) giving birth (via natural conception or the help of medical science), (2) adoption, or (3) childfree living. Only you can determine what your specific needs are and what options are available in your situation. None of the choices is an easy answer, but all outcomes can be rewarding.

Ending the Struggle

Only some of you will end your infertility struggle by successfully delivering a child, but through resolution, all of you can find your own means of satisfaction and a sense of peace.

This chapter describes the three ways in which couples end their infertility struggle—by giving birth, adopting, or remaining childfree. Each of these endings brings with it its own joys, but also its own stresses that need to be addressed. Whatever your particular ending turns out to be, you can be assured there is life after infertility, and a very happy one at that!

Giving Birth—The Pregnant Infertile Woman

Regardless of how you have conceived—normally or through medical technology—the experience of pregnancy after infertility can be wonderful. For some, however, it can also be a little disconcerting. Although you may have assumed that once a positive pregnancy test arrives, the slate will be wiped clean and you will live happily ever after, it isn't always so simple. As one infertile woman said, "If I ever do get pregnant, I think I will still feel and be infertile; it's like being an alcoholic. It lives with you forever."

Many find, when learning they are pregnant after an extended time fighting infertility, that there are no fireworks—the long-awaited dream is full of joy, but it is tempered by fear and mistrust. Having lived with frustration and disappointment for so long, they are fearful that something will go wrong yet again.

I had a very easy, comfortable pregnancy but could not

*enjoy it—I worried constantly. I never really believed
that I would bear a child. Even when my waters broke,
I didn't really comprehend what was happening. My
long, very painful labor was easier to deal with—it
was too harsh to deny. In retrospect, I have very happy
memories of labor and delivery but feel somewhat sad
about my pregnancy. I wish I could have enjoyed it
more.*

The first trimester may be especially anxiety-provoking because of the possibility of miscarriage. Many, however, are on pins and needles throughout the entire pregnancy, refusing to believe in a successful outcome until it happens. Anxiety flourishes because the stakes are so high.

A lot depends, of course, on how long you struggled with infertility before conceiving, but it can be difficult facing reality after having idealized the pregnancy-birth event. Those who have experienced the nine months know it is not always a blissful time, but you can't tell that to an infertile woman—she doesn't want to hear it. Her dreams have never included feelings of nausea, episodes of vomiting, panic attacks over spotting, bloatedness, or excessive weight gain. Not everyone experiences these symptoms, but they are common. Although you may have intellectually acknowledged these possibilities during your infertile days, the chances are you fantasized a rosy, happier time. When others complained during their pregnancies, you probably said—and meant it—that you would put up with any amount of misery just to be in their shoes. But now you are finally pregnant, and you are feeling less than terrific—but how can you complain? Although many are disturbed by these feelings, you should try not to be too hard on yourself for not always feeling wonderful and not always reveling in your pregnancy.

A further quandary ensues, if you lose the support and camaraderie you had with your infertile friends. You know all too well how hard it is for them to be around a pregnant woman, but losing your closeness with them leaves you feeling stranded. Your fertile friends will be happy for you, but they cannot understand your vulnerability and your worries. It can be a lonely situation, far from what you had expected. Surprisingly, even now you have to face insensitivity from the fertile world: "See, I told you you'd get pregnant. I don't know why you worried so much!" or "Now you know nothing was wrong with you!"

Delivery is seldom easy, but, again, in the fantasies of the infertile, the experience was transformed into something blissful. It may be disappointing if your dream of natural childbirth or the togetherness and joy of delivery do not come to pass as expected. The fact is that both pregnancy and delivery, for a first-timer (whether or not after an infertility struggle), tend to be arduous. Barbara Eck Menning notes, too, that some studies estimate that cesarean sections are performed twice as often among women with previous infertility problems than among others. Their pregnancies are considered exceptionally valuable, and physicians do not want to risk anything happening.

In sum, the infertile woman who becomes pregnant expects perfection because that's the stuff dreams are made of. When the reality of pregnancy, delivery, and parenting sets in, the disappointment can make you feel guilty for not appreciating what you have. Try not to worry—your feelings are normal. Just remember all those months or years of infertility treatment, and what you're going through now will seem like a breeze.

Adoption

To an Adopted

I
Did not plant you,
True.
But when
The season is done—
When the alternate
Prayers for sun
And for rain
Are counted—
When the pain
Of Weeding
And the pride
Of Watching
Are through—

Then
I will hold you
High,
A shining sheaf
Above the thousand
Seeds grown wild.

Not my planting,
But by heaven
My harvest—
My own child.

> — Carol Lynn Pearson
> Walnut Creek, California
> from *The Search*

Pursuing adoption is, for most, a lengthy and difficult emotional process that begins long before that first telephone call to an adoption agency or the first inquiry to a lawyer. Early in an infertility workup, when hope runs high and one needs to deny the possibility of a serious problem, any mention of adoption may elicit feelings of fear as well as hostility toward those who raise the subject. You may even have pitied someone you knew who had to adopt and thought of the option as a last resort.

When friends of ours adopted, it was a very uneasy time for me. It was two years before we would eventually make that step ourselves and, at the time, adoption was a taboo subject—it wasn't going to happen to us. In visiting our friends shortly after the baby's arrival, I felt happiness for them but had a very disconcerting feeling. Their failure at having a biological child was hitting too close to home and I wasn't ready to face it. On the way home, I remarked to my husband, "It's just not the same as having your own. They don't seem as excited as they should be." I realize now that that feeling was a projection of my own anxiety at the moment and my worry that one day we'd "have" to adopt, too. In reality, our friends were thrilled, just as we were two years later at the

arrival of our adopted daughter. It just took time to
reach that point—a process that couldn't be speeded up
but had to take its course.

As infertility treatments come and go and unsuccessful months pass by, perceptions change, often in small, unidentifiable ways. All of a sudden, one day, you may realize that you can discuss the topic of adoption without feeling pangs or rushing to change the subject. Denial has changed to curiosity and interest.

Frequent Worries

Adoption, although common, is still different from the norm and carries with it many emotional issues. A frequent fear is: "Will I be able to love this child as much as I'd love one that we produced?" As one man said,

I'm just not sure. I'd like to believe that I would love
an adopted child as much as my own, but I'm not sure
I trust myself. I'm afraid that in a moment of future
anger, I might say something very hurtful to him like "I
wish we'd never adopted you." It scares me that I might
always have some doubts, perhaps deep inside but still
there.

What people often do not understand is that the bonding that occurs between a parent and baby is an "emotional glue" that transcends the blood relationship. Your feelings for your child—whether adopted or biological—can be equally intense. It may be hard to recognize this, however, until you have experienced it.

Another factor when considering adoption is the need to confront your feelings about hitting a genetic dead end. The loss of genetic immortality is, for many, hard to accept. And some people, too, fear that an adopted child will ultimately abandon them in favor of the biological parents. Most adopted children, however, never seek out their birthparents. Scotland, for example, has a national registry from which adoptive individuals can obtain information regarding their biological parents, and yet a ten-year study revealed that only 1.5 out of every 1,000 adult adoptees sought out their original birth certificate.[1] Even when reunions do occur, in most instances the experience only strengthens the relationship between the child and the adoptive parents. Being a good parent has nothing to do with being able to conceive and deliver a child.

Another worry for some is the belief that adopted children have more emotional difficulties than biological children and that you are asking for trouble if you choose this route. Again, the fact is that studies have revealed no difference between adopted and natural children regarding their mental health.[2] Being adopted, of course, is a significant issue for children, and some may experience feelings of abandonment, depression, or anger. The crucial factor, though, is not whether these responses occur but how they are dealt with by family members. Actually, it has been noted that couples who have faced and worked through infertility are often especially well equipped to become excellent adoptive parents. Because they have effectively confronted their own loss, they are likely to better understand their child's feelings of loss and abandonment, and can help the youngster to deal constructively with these painful emotions. All children must face traumas or disappointments in their lives at some time, whether they live in adopted or biological families. It is the manner in which the child is raised and the feelings experienced in the family that will determine the outcome.

Some couples considering adoption worry that their families will disapprove and even reject them or the adopted child, especially in the case of a youngster with a different racial or ethnic background. As mentioned earlier in this book, you should remember that extended family members also need time to assimilate your decision to adopt. If you have finally chosen adoption after a lengthy emotional process and then suddenly dump this decision in your parents' lap with no warning, it is unfair to expect instant understanding. Make sure you give them some time to adjust, also.

Still another common concern may be that you will adopt and then later conceive. How will you feel then about the adopted child? Although the common belief that those who adopt are sure to get pregnant is untrue, one may still worry that a new form of treatment or a new understanding of the reproductive problem will later lead to conception. One adoptive parent had this to say:

In the years prior to adopting, my worst fear was that I would finally decide to adopt, only to get pregnant a

few months later. Implicit in this fear was the
assumption that I'd consider our adopted child a
"mistake" and wish we'd had the patience to wait just a
little longer. Well, we did make that decision to adopt
and our son is now four years old. Although I never did
become pregnant, it's hard for me to believe that I ever
had that worry in the first place. Just looking at my
son is enough to know I could never love another child,
even one I biologically produced, more than him. I
really had no understanding, at that time, about the
intensity of a parent's love for a child, adopted or
natural.

Infertile couples often feel pressure to adopt, especially if efforts to conceive have continued for a long time. Friends may tire of your problem and question why you don't adopt if you want a baby so badly; others who have already adopted may enthusiastically recommend the option for you. Sometimes one partner is ready to adopt, but the other is not, which can create a strain. But you should never try to force yourself to be comfortable with adoption, if inside the idea is disturbing. This is not a time for selflessness. Negative feelings may eventually change, but you should not adopt until you are ready. Some anxiety and questioning will exist throughout the adoption process—that's normal. But if excitement and eager anticipation are not your overriding emotions, the time has not yet come for you to take this crucial step. You must face honestly any doubts you have before proceeding.

There are two basic tasks that must be largely accomplished before proceeding with an actual placement. First, you must have faced and accepted your feelings about being infertile. That means working through your disappointment and mourning your inability to produce a biological child. You have spent a long time trying to conquer your infertility, but it wasn't successful. Those painful feeling cannot be denied. Second, you must accept the reality of adoption. It is different from biological parenthood—not worse, just different. You must be willing to acknowledge those differences. If you continue to fantasize about the biological child you do not have or you are uncomfortable with the many emotional issues that will crop up once adoption takes place (such as telling others about the adoption and answering their questions, accepting the reality of the child's birthparents, eventually discussing adoption with the child), you may need additional time and help to deal with this option. Patricia Johnston, in *An Adopter's Advocate*, has an excellent discussion of these issues.

Deciding to Adopt

If you do decide that adoption is a real option for you, the worry becomes not "will we adopt?" but "how will we adopt?" and "will we find a baby?" Prior to the 1970s, adoption was a viable solution to infertility. Healthy babies of different races were more accessible to the childless couple owing to numerous factors—less use of birth control, fewer abortions, and a higher percentage of single women who chose to relinquish their babies for adoption.

Over the past two decades, the situation has changed. Although approximately one of every six infants born in the United States is delivered by a single woman, half of these women now keep their children. Adolescents, in particular, are increasingly choosing to do this. Thus, the picture may seem bleak when you first make inquiries, especially if you are seeking a healthy, white newborn. But perseverance will pay off. There are a number of books on adoption that can help you during your efforts to find a child. Two of these are *The Penguin Adoption Handbook* by Edmund Blair Bolles and *The Adoption Resource Book* by Lois Gilman (see the Bibliography for others).

At the beginning, others who have adopted can be a major source of encouragement. Make an effort to learn everything possible about their experience. Be willing to share your goal with others because that is how information is obtained. You will find a grapevine of adoption suggestions that is invaluable, and you may be surprised to learn how many adoptive parents and children are around. Pursue every resource—finding a child is often by word of mouth. If you understand all the options—agency, independent, and foreign placements; special needs children—you can select the one that is most comfortable for you.

For some, adoption goes smoothly and quickly with their first efforts, whereas for others there can be long waits and painful disappointments. The latter possibility is, unfortunately, more likely. Whatever you do, though, don't give up in the face of frustration and early failures.

Before discussing the different types of adoption, I want to mention the issue of pursuing adoption and pregnancy at the same time. This is commonly done by older couples who feel that time is against them and don't want to leave any stone unturned. Also, with waiting lists being lengthy, it only makes sense that many will want to get their names into an agency while still undergoing medical treatment. Home studies generally do not occur immediately, so you may just sit on the waiting list. Just a few words of caution are important, however. First, some adoption agencies are not pleased with this approach because they want a definite commitment from a couple. In these cases, you will have to decide what to say during the interviews, when asked about ongoing medical efforts; only you can make that choice. Many other agencies, however, are beginning to recognize that a continuing quest for biological parenthood does not preclude adoption or affect it negatively. Second, some forms of adoption can proceed very quickly, such as independent placements, so be careful about starting those inquiries if you are not yet certain about your readiness to adopt. It can be distressing to find suddenly that a baby is available and you are not emotionally prepared for it. Third, actively pursuing both pregnancy and adoption can be stressful. Don't set yourself up for excessive chaos and strain by scheduling significant conflicting events in close proximity—say, meeting with an adoption agency one day and attempting in vitro fertilization the next. And, finally, if the home study has been completed and you are told that adoption will soon be possible, it is important now to focus your thoughts and efforts on that decision. You will need time to prepare emotionally for your adopted child and to ensure that grieving for the loss of the biological baby has been done. All of this is not to say that proceeding in two directions at the same time can't be done. It can—but it may be taxing. You must explore your feelings very carefully.

If you decide at a later point to reenter medical treatment, this by itself does not signify unresolved feelings about adoption or failure to bond to your adopted child. Many have come to realize that their primary desire is to be parents, but that they would still like to take advantage of any progress made in medical technology. A couple may, therefore, adopt happily but decide to pursue a new treatment for biological parenthood in years to come.

Agency Placement

Initial efforts at trying to adopt through an agency can be very discouraging. There is nothing worse than calling a few agencies, only to be told that their lists are closed, there is a waiting period of five years, you don't meet their religious requirements, and/or you are over their age limit. Unfortunately, relatively few babies are now available through adoption agencies, and the waiting time, even if you meet the agency's requirements, will average three to six years. You must be prepared for some frustration and be willing to persevere in your efforts to find an agency that can meet your needs.

You can compile a list of names by checking the Yellow Pages of telephone directories, calling your state's Department of Social Services, contacting RESOLVE, or attending meetings of adoptive parents' groups in your area. When you call an agency, ask about the availability of children, basic requirements, length of waiting lists, home visit and placement procedures, and fees. Be careful not to get your hopes up too high, however, if an agency invites you to meet with its staff. It may just be an informational meeting for large numbers of people. Some couples have found these early agency interviews to be a very trying experience, especially when they are asked to turn their lives inside out for perusal, only to learn in the end that very few babies are available.

PROS AND CONS OF AGENCY
ADOPTION

There are advantages and disadvantages to agency adoption as there are to other adoption options. In agency placement, the birthmother (or birthparents) places the child with an agency, which then selects a couple from their lists to receive it. You may make some initial input regarding your particular needs, but the agency makes the match. Both birthparents and adoptive parents usually remain anonymous, although some agencies are beginning to offer opportunities for limited contact. Anonymity will be comfortable for some, whereas others may find it to be a disadvantage.

An additional factor is that agencies often place the baby first in foster care before arranging a permanent adoption. This is a drawback if you want to adopt an infant directly after birth. It is an advantage, though, in that birthparents must relinquish custody *before* the child is placed with adoptive parents. You will probably not even know a child is available for you until the placement is definite, which usually ensures that attempts will not be made to reclaim the child. Thus, adopting through an agency is the safest avenue to take.

UNDERSTANDING THE HOME STUDY

Some prospective adoptive couples find themselves intimidated by adoption workers during a home study. Being scrutinized unquestionably can produce uncomfortable feelings. But recognize that the agencies are serving as advocates for the child. If you can accept their position, it may help you feel less threatened.

Agencies will want to carefully determine how well you have accepted your infertility. They will also evaluate your marriage to make sure it is healthy and stable and will inquire into your support system—the family and friends who will be available for understanding and help. Agencies like to think of their home studies less as an investigation and more as a means of helping a couple assess their feelings and motivations for adoption. The procedure can be useful, and in many cases close relationships eventually develop between the couple and the adoption worker.

Our positive feelings about our worker, about going to see her (we always turned it into an outing), and about the content of our home study interviews enabled us to view adoption in a very positive way. When we received a surprise call that our daughter was arriving in less than twenty-four hours, we went into a wonderful, hysterical, unforgettable whirlwind. Her arrival was fantastic! Our relationship with our adoption worker has remained very special. We take her out to dinner each year on our daughter's birthday, and she and her family come for a barbecue each summer. She remains our most beloved magician!

SPECIAL NEEDS CHILDREN

In considering agency placement, you might also be interested in the adoption of special needs children. A readily available alternative, it requires a very special kind of parent. These children include those with severe physical or emotional handicaps, those who are mentally retarded, siblings who should remain together, and older children who have often been through difficult family situations. Those who investigate this option should carefully examine their own needs, their experience and expertise and, most important, the needs of the child, which may be many.

Adopting a special needs child can be extremely rewarding, but it is a far cry from adopting a healthy newborn. The youngsters, for example, may have trouble relating to others because of their chaotic or sad histories. Adoptive parents often are not prepared for these children's negative attitudes or disruptive behavior. The instability of their previous relationships rarely provides them with positive self-images or self-confidence. And such youngsters often question the permanency of the new situation and may seriously test the relationship.

Many parents feel that because they have so much love to give, their love will cure all. This is not always the case, however. Couples who pursue this option must recognize that it will probably take a long time for a sense of real trust and closeness to evolve—and that an enormous degree of patience will be necessary. If you are not prepared for this problem, you may find the experience frustrating and very disappointing. Carefully evaluate your expectations before embarking on the adoption of a special needs child.

LEGAL-RISK ADOPTION

Legal-risk adoption, also called foster-adoption, is another option for the infertile couple. This involves children who are presently in need of foster care but who, it is expected, will be available for adoption as soon as the birthparents relinquish their parental rights. Often, babies and toddlers are available for this kind of placement.

The main problem here is that it may take considerable time before the child is legally free to be adopted, and during that period, birthparents sometimes change their minds about relinquishment. As long as a child is in foster care, the birthparents also have the right to visit. This situation, then, is risky and anxiety provoking, but if you can handle the uncertainty, it is worth looking into. The cost of this option can also be much less than other forms of adoption.

Independent Placement

Independent or private placement occurs when a couple makes an independent arrangement with a birthmother, often through an intermediary (usually a physician or attorney). It is legal in forty-four states, with the understanding that the birthmother places the baby in the care of a particular couple or single adult who pays related medical and legal expenses.

It is important to understand that adopting independently is *not* black-market adoption or baby-selling, although often the line between them is blurred. Baby-selling involves an individual (birthmother, attorney, or other intermediary) financially profiting from the adoption of a child. Many think that an independent placement is always very expensive, but that is not necessarily so— arrangements often involve only basic medical and legal costs.

THE ADVANTAGES OF INDEPENDENT PLACEMENT

Edmund Bolles, in *The Penguin Adoption Handbook*, writes, "There is no baby shortage. The shortages in the adoption world are shortages of information and organization."[3] This is especially true of independent adoption placements. The adoption scene has dramatically changed in recent years, and single women are no longer turning to agencies to place their babies for adoption but instead are maintaining control by making their own private arrangements. You may find a baby that is available to adopt through independent placement if you are willing to put some effort into a search and if you are emotionally able to take some risks. An advantage of this method is that you can avoid the long waits so typical of agency placements.

There are many innovative ways for couples to initiate an independent placement. Some write personal letters or have printed a letter that can be copied and widely distributed. Sometimes they advertise in newspapers throughout the country. To some, the idea of advertising for a baby may be repugnant, but if it results in your adoption of a healthy infant, my feeling is what difference does it make? Contact RESOLVE or an adoptive parents group in your area to get further ideas and referrals to competent attorneys.

If independent placements are not allowed in your state, a procedure called *identified adoption* may be an option for you. This happens when a couple becomes aware of a birthmother who is interested in having her baby adopted by independent placement. The couple contacts an adoption agency that agrees to oversee the adoption and will provide its services to the birthmother, child, and couple. This would include counseling, a home study, a medical evaluation of the baby, and necessary paperwork. Many agencies will not accommodate such an arrangement, so you may need to persevere in looking for one that offers this program.

THE RISKS OF INDEPENDENT PLACEMENTS

Private placements are clearly riskier than those made through an agency, but there are ways to reduce the risks and protect yourself. Listed here are a few guidelines. Refer to the books and articles listed in the Bibliography for others.

1. Understand the laws in your state pertaining to independent arrangements.

2. Procure a reputable attorney who is experienced in adoption.

3. Be sure that payments include only the lawyer's fee and the birthmother's expenses, although the latter will vary depending on whether it includes her medical expenses, living costs, her attorney's fees, or travel arrangements. Be careful of requests for excessive amounts.

4. Attorneys usually recommend that some anonymity be maintained—not giving your full name, home address, or place of work. Keeping this in mind, decide on the amount or type of contact you want. Some communication, whether by telephone, letter (perhaps sent through an intermediary), or in person, seems advantageous in that it can help reassure both parties of the other's motivations and interest. Too much contact, though, may encourage a strong sense of rivalry or an inability to separate once the adoption has taken place.

5. Either you or your intermediary must be sure to obtain medical information regarding the birthparents and their families as well as other relevant history.

6. Always have the baby thoroughly examined by a pediatrician in the hospital or while still in the birthmother's care.

The riskiest aspect of an independent placement, of course, is the fact that until parental rights are terminated, the birthparents can reclaim the child. We have all heard horror stories about birthparents changing their minds, and it is easy to be frightened by the possibilities for heartache. But the successes far outnumber the disasters, and if you can weather the potential storms, the baby in your arms at the end will be worth every bit of worry and struggle. Again, only you can decide whether an independent placement is worth the risk.

Initially, I wanted nothing at all to do with adopting privately. I had heard horrendous situations from others, like the birthmother just disappearing during her ninth month or the baby being born with serious medical problems, and I didn't want to chance having that kind of experience. Going the agency route, though, proved to be so frustrating that when a private arrangement became available, we decided to risk it. To my surprise, the whole process went beautifully, although I know we were very lucky.

International Placement

International adoption began after World War II and has steadily increased ever since, with a surge in recent years. Over the past decade, more than thirty thousand babies have been adopted from foreign countries, most commonly Korea, India, Colombia, and El Salvador. This is almost a 200 percent increase during the past ten years.[4]

Despite frequent and extensive red tape, many couples have chosen this form of adoption because of its high degree of success. Some of the advantages of international placement are that infants are more readily available from other countries and waiting times can be significantly less. Not surprisingly, though, the length of time is increasing as more and more couples select this route.

In beginning your efforts toward international adoption, it is very helpful to speak with other couples who have adopted children from foreign countries. Attending an adoptive parents' group can be an excellent start for making contacts and learning how to best pursue this form of adoption. The procedures may seem complicated, but there are definite steps to follow. The Latin America Parents Association has available a brief summary describing the process (see Resources). Another free booklet on the procedures of foreign adoption, *The Immigration of Adopted and Prospective Adoptive Children*, can be obtained from the Outreach Program, U.S. Immigration and Naturalization Service, 425 I Street N.W., Room 6230, Washington, DC 20536. Other groups to contact include the Open Door Society, OURS, Inc., and Families Adopting Children Everywhere (F.A.C.E.).

You can also write or call agencies and ask what countries they are involved with, what kinds of children are available, the number of placements they make, and their waiting period.

For foreign adoptions that are handled privately, the process usually begins by your contacting an intermediary, often an attorney, in the United States or by directly communicating with an individual in the foreign country who arranges placements (a physician, the head of an orphanage, an attorney, or a social worker). The paperwork and red tape can be voluminous, but eventually it gets done as attested to by the high number of successful placements.

COMMON ANXIETIES

It is not unusual, along the way, to feel some anxiety and perhaps ambivalence—"Are we doing the right thing?" and "Are we ready for this?" It may just be the reality of taking on the responsibility for parenthood or it may be that you are having second thoughts about adopting a child from another ethnic background. Discuss these feelings *now* with your spouse and others close to you. Adoption workers can also be of great assistance in exploring these feelings. Being a parent is hard enough, but the added burden of critical social attitudes when adopting a foreign child can make the job even more difficult. It is crucial that you both have secure self-images and are confident of your decision.

HANDLING SOCIAL REACTIONS

Community and family reactions to the adoption of a child from a different racial and cultural background will vary, but adoptive parents must be ready to face both criticism and insensitive comments. Although it would be helpful if everyone reacted with acceptance and support, there will unfortunately be those who disapprove or are hostile. Both parents and children may have to put up with the stares and questioning of others, even when they are not ill-natured.

EXPLORING YOUR OWN PREJUDICES

Prospective adoptive parents must also be willing to examine closely their own feelings and attitudes. Not many of us grow up without some amount of prejudice, even if only very subtle. A child from another country will be arriving with his or her own racial, ethnic, and cultural background. If you find these differences to be exciting and interesting, that's terrific. But many people are overwhelmed by anxiety and fear when confronted with a situation that is "different," and you will have to deal with this in yourself and in others. Remember that everyone loves a cute baby. But that cute baby will eventually grow older, looking dissimilar to you in all likelihood. It is important to give this some serious thought. Will you be able totally to accept that adorable baby as an older child and adult?

Adoptive parents cannot and should not deny the ethnic background of their children. It is part of their identity and they must eventually be able to assimilate both their adopted family and their biological origins. As adoptive parents, therefore, you must be willing to develop an understanding of your child's heritage and to convey your acceptance of that background, so the child feels security and pride.

The Adoption Experience

Worries about adopting are numerous, even after a definite decision has been made and you have begun arrangements privately or through an agency. Awaiting adoption is unlike the preparation time involved in nine months of pregnancy. Even if you have made independent plans and have a due date to anticipate, the experience is far more uncertain than knowing life is inside you and feeling all the changes. With adoption, nothing concrete happens—you must simply wait.

Once again, you are not in control—the recurring theme of infertility. Agency investigations may especially rekindle those angry, frustrated feelings. There may be tears, and lots of them, as the anxiety grows. Each ring of the telephone means another breathless moment.

I was terrified the birthmother would change her mind.
As her due date came closer, I could barely control my

anxiety and felt totally helpless. Since it was a private placement, I had her phone number and could call anytime, but I didn't want to overwhelm her with daily calls, which is what I felt like doing. I busied myself with preparations for the baby and desperately tried not to think of the worst.

People handle the waiting period in very different ways, regardless of the type of adoptive placement. Some move ahead and furnish a nursery, thus making the situation more real; others fear the possibility of arrangements falling through and refuse to prepare until the last minute. Some secretly make their own quiet plans. You may find yourself cautiously venturing into baby stores, lingering over a little outfit, and perhaps hiding away a few small items for that special day. It can be very hard to admit openly your growing excitement, for fear it will not come true. When disappointment has become such a routine part of your life, it is difficult to turn from pessimism to confidence and optimism. Some find that, while awaiting adoption, they are particularly uncomfortable around pregnant women, whereas others find that their decision to adopt brings an easing of the tensions.

Both my sister and sister-in-law delivered babies two months before we adopted our son. At the time of those births, we hadn't yet made the adoption arrangement, so we were sitting in limbo, anxiously making inquiries all over. Still, the fact that we had finally decided to adopt was the only thing that helped me face the births of my two nieces. Had we been continuing to struggle with unsuccessful infertility treatments, I question how I would have survived that time. Instead, my own ability to finally see a light at the end of the tunnel made me able to share in my family's happiness.

Eventually, that all-important and long-awaited telephone call does come—YOU ARE GOING TO BE PARENTS! Most who adopt find that the ecstasy of that phone call and first holding the baby in their arms is beyond compare. Many describe it as love at first sight.

*Somehow all the worries just disappear when you hold
that baby for the first time. In our situation, we
learned, just a half hour before getting our son, that he
had developed some feeding problems in the hospital,
was vomiting, and might have a serious problem. Yet,
when I set eyes on him, I didn't have one moment of
regret about adopting him, with or without medical
problems. He was ours, I adored him, and that's all that
counted. Certainly, I wanted him to be healthy, but not
once did I think, "Oh no, we've got a defective baby."*

Whether or not you believe in fate, the experience of adopting a
child can be so intensely felt that it is easy to feel that the match was
"just meant to be."

Postadoption Blues

Regardless of the time you have spent fighting infertility or waiting
to adopt, the experience of being a parent through adoption is
abrupt and overwhelming. Although it is obvious that the arrival of
an adopted child in your home will radically change your lives, just
as the birth of a biological baby does, many adoptive parents, especially mothers, fail to realize that they are likely to experience some
down feelings, too. Don't be surprised by feelings of anxiety, leth-
argy, irritability, or depression—they are normal responses to a sudden upheaval in your life. The abrupt change in your life-style and
the tremendous responsibility you've taken on can be a little overwhelming. Dreams rarely prepare you for the reality of this experience.

*For the first six months, I was on Cloud 9 and probably
functioning on nervous energy. I was thrilled to be a
mother and often had to pinch myself to prove it was
real. Gradually, though, I began to feel exhausted,
anxious, and generally rundown. I convinced myself
that something terrible must be happening to my body
and went for a physical examination, only to learn
that I was in top-notch shape. Only after getting that
clean bill of health did I acknowledge just how much*

my life had changed. It had been a complete
transformation and was finally taking its toll on me
emotionally.

Although the hormonal changes that accompany the birth of a baby will not occur, the environmental stresses will be just as real. Both parents will feel in a state of disequilibrium as they adjust to the impact of a new member of the family. Routines will drastically change, and it will take time for relationships to adapt.

Another aspect of this postadoption time which may be disconcerting is that you are likely to receive a barrage of questions and comments about adoption. Many adoptive parents find this to be exciting and interesting, while others may feel uncomfortable, uncertain how to respond or how much to tell. Personally, I found everyone's interest to be thrilling, not intrusive, and I enjoyed sharing the details of the adoption. However, everyone reacts differently and only you can decide how to handle each situation. Remember, though, that people are naturally curious about adoption and that questions usually stem from caring and interest, not just nosiness. How you respond to others will probably reflect your inner feelings about adoption and how comfortable you are with your decision. This is a time, though, when painful feelings about your infertility will normally appear again—so don't be surprised by them. With so much discussion about adoption and the reality of a child in your home, it's no wonder that these feelings are surfacing.

Unwelcome comments are likely to continue after adoption, just as they did during your infertility struggle. One common remark is "Well, you certainly took the easy way out." You can ignore such comments, take them with a grain of salt, or respond with the truth (e.g., "Five years to have a baby isn't my idea of the easy way out"). Again, though, try to remember that these remarks generally arise out of others' discomfort with adoption and their need to make light of the situation.

Adopting an older child or one from a foreign country will present unique concerns. In the case of an older child, you may find yourself disappointed if friends or relatives seem less enthralled than you imagined or would have liked. Try to be realistic in your expectations.

Another significant factor, during this first year after the child has arrived, is that it can take six months to a year before the adoption is actually finalized. Home visits from an adoption agency may continue, both with agency and independent placements, and anxiety can remain high, as couples feel their ability to be good parents is still being evaluated. Those who have privately adopted often worry that a birthparent will change her mind before the finalization or that she will suddenly appear on the doorstep. These are disconcerting but real issues in the adoption process. My own feeling about this, having lived through the experience, is that there is little point in dwelling on these worries because there is nothing to be done. Luckily, the time and energy required for a new child helps keep you occupied and less focused on negative thoughts.

Adoption, in the end, can be the answer to your dreams, but it is not an easy road to travel, nor can anyone guarantee a positive outcome. Of course, the same is true for those having biological children.

Another point: adoption does not resolve your feelings about infertility. That you must do on your own. Adoption, however, creates the wonderful opportunity for parenthood that eludes so many people for so many years, and it can feel like the greatest of miracles. In conclusion, remember this admonition, which says it all: "Families are not born; they are created and developed through years of patience and love."[4]

Childfree Living

A third option for infertile couples is to remain childfree. The couple makes a deliberate decision to continue life without children, with their feelings about their infertility resolved. Such a choice is far different from that of couples who continue efforts to have children, forever feeling their childlessness to be a detriment or loss. Choosing to remain childfree must be exactly that—a choice, even though this may not be what the couple originally wanted.

After years of trying to conceive, even the suggestion of childfree living as an option may seem either foreign or very frightening. Your response may be, "That's a ridiculous idea! Why do you think we've been driving ourselves crazy for all these years?" Even though the choice is rejected by many, it can be the right alternative for some.

Understanding Your Motivations to Have a Child

Probably the majority of fertile couples, who easily had children, never fully assessed their motivations, readiness, or desire to be parents. People often have children because it seems to be the thing to do. Friends are starting families, parents want grandchildren, and everyone concerned expects it. If there is one positive thing that infertility accomplishes, however, it is to force people to examine themselves and their lives, and consider carefully what they need and want.

It is possible that some people are at first uncertain about becoming parents but make the effort anyway, only to be confronted with their infertility. In the process of fighting the problem, they may forget their early doubts and be drawn into a battle to regain control of their fertility—only now not so much because they desire children but because they want it to be a choice. Only you can assess what the infertility struggle has been for you—an effort to have a baby or a battle for control with God, nature, or medicine. Acknowledging the latter to yourself, after years of infertility, can be very difficult, but it may be an eye-opening admission that will help you move forward.

Culturally, married couples are expected to have offspring. It can be hard to go against the norm, although perhaps it's becoming easier. Many fertile couples today make a conscious decision not to have children and take irrevocable medical steps to ensure they don't. Among professional couples, childfree living is not rare or even unusual. Despite this, however, many people still assume you will be unfulfilled without children, and they might even judge you to be selfish or immature. Merle Bombardieri, however, who has written extensively on the childfree alternative (see RESOLVE publications "Childfree Decision-Making" and the *The Baby Decision*) states

> *Research does not confirm this stereotype. Extensive psychosocial studies have found childfree couples to be just as happy as couples with children. And contrary to the stereotype of selfishness, a high percentage of childfree people are teachers, social workers, or people who spend their weekends doing volunteer work with children or for a social cause. It's far more common for*

selfish, immature people to have children for selfish, immature reasons.[5]

Often, a major worry may be the pressure from friends or relatives who fail to understand why you even consider this option, let alone follow through on it. Not recognizing the soul-searching that infertility can catalyze, others may respond, "How could you put yourselves through all that suffering and then decide you don't want kids?" Even other infertile couples will sometimes be unable to understand your considering this option. Actually, they may be threatened by your choice because it touches upon their own conflicts.

Many people love children, but when they think it through, they realize their lives are not compatible with being parents. These individuals may find their relationships with others' children rewarding, or they may pursue involvement with youngsters through a different avenue, like teaching, coaching sports, or being a Scout leader.

Some people simply do not want to parent another person's biological child through adoption or feel they could not deal with the problems involved. When evaluating your motivations, you may discover that the experience of pregnancy and childbirth, or the desire to carry on family traits, were really the primary aims of your efforts. Thus, adoption would fail to meet your needs and a childfree life may be the better alternative. Some, after years of infertility treatment, may simply be exhausted. Adoption brings with it a whole new set of issues, and you may feel too worn out to start another struggle. Adoption then would be a new chore, not a means of resolution.

The Benefits of Living Childfree

Many people have misconceptions about what a decision for childfree living actually means. As with any of the outcomes discussed in this book, the choice of remaining childfree means ending the roller coaster of emotions you have been through. It means that you can stop treatment, stop being frustrated, and stop waiting, watching, and wondering. It means you can move on to living again.

My husband and I have come to accept our situation.

We've grieved through the loss of our dream and have made the decision to be childfree. I now have an inner peace and outer excitement about life that I haven't had in eight years. Since I now have control over my life, it will go on with meaning and purpose. The door has been closed on eight years of unhappiness, and a new door is opening because of this decision. We've finally brought the entire situation to a conclusion.[6]

When you are chasing the dream of a baby, it is easy to forget that life has the potential for many other dreams and fulfillments. Deciding on a childfree life leaves room to explore the endless possibilities of career, travel, recreation, hobbies, and togetherness as a couple. Although those who choose to have children may experience rewards and feel no regret, they may often feel a sense of loss over the opportunities that childfree living offers. It is crucial, however, for both partners, should they choose the childfree alternative, to feel they can happily fill up their lives with work and other interests. If one partner pursues a successful career, but the other has little to replace the parenting function, unhappy consequences are likely.

Common Fears and Worries

One of the biggest fears people express when considering a childfree life is that they will regret this decision in their older years and end up being lonely and miserable. Merle Bombardieri, states that "children are no insurance policy against loneliness in old age."[7] She notes several elements that affect loneliness in later years, including health, income, ability to maintain old friends and find new ones, the extent to which an extended family network has been built, the ability to be assertive in asking for help or companionship, and the ability to maintain old interests and find new ones. Children are a factor in one's adjustment to old age, but they are by no means the only one.

People also worry that when they die, they will have nothing to leave behind. The truth is that children are not the only ones who remember you, nor are they the only means of establishing continuity or everlasting memory. Being a mentor to others in your field of work, working to change or improve your community, or sharing your creative talents are just a few obvious ways of establishing immortality besides parenthood.

Making the Choice

The choice to remain childfree, then, is not an easy or quick decision, and you may not be supported in it by others in your life. Your age and the life-style of your friends will most likely have a strong effect on the degree of difficulty you have in pursuing this option. Certainly, it will be harder if your friends are all involved in raising families and you feel out of the mainstream. As time passes, though, children grow, and others will find themselves returning to a way of life similar to yours.

What happens if you and your spouse disagree about what to do? It is not unusual for one partner to be comfortable with the prospect of a childfree life, while the other is seriously considering adoption or donor insemination. Needless to say, this can cause tremendous conflict and heartache. As noted earlier in the chapter "Infertility and the Couple," it is important not to panic at the first signs of disagreement. Often, time is needed for each partner to understand better his own feelings and to learn more about his spouse's point of view.

> *I wanted to adopt, but Phil didn't. I remember our driving home from an adoption meeting and comparing reactions. While I was happily fantasizing about our adopted family, Phil was concluding that adoption was not for him. He just wasn't sure he could fully commit himself to accept and raise a child who was not his own flesh and blood. I was in a dilemma—how could I adopt if my husband was against it? Suddenly, I was very lonely. Infertility treatment had brought us together, but the adoption issue set us at odds with each other. It was very isolating. We resolved the conflict by going together to a counselor who was very helpful. It turned out that I had never really let go of the hope that I would get pregnant. I had some grief work to do before I could give the childfree choice a consideration. Counseling enabled us to renew our commitment to each other and*

to our marriage. Only after grieving and renewing my
commitment to Phil was I ready to consider and to
accept remaining childfree.[8]

As with any of the options for resolution, mourning the loss of
that biologically conceived child must take place before decision
making. With the childfree choice, however, you must also mourn
the fantasied adopted child. Those who do not grieve will continue
to feel a sense of regret and will probably be unable to make the
most of their childfree decision. Even when mourning has occurred,
the pain of infertility may occasionally surface, but it will be a lesser
pain and short-lived, unlike the anguish of the past. No matter how
well thought out your decision may be and how certain you feel
about it, there are bound to be future moments of doubt and questioning. Life is full of crossroads when difficult choices must be made
as to which direction to follow. It is normal to experience moments
of "what if . . .?"

And remember that a childfree decision is not irrevocable (unless you have chosen to have a tubal ligation or vasectomy). You can
change your mind at some point in the future and resume treatment
or pursue adoption. Again, that is your choice.

In conclusion, the value of and reward from resolution is what
you make of it. If you select a childfree life and then treat it as a
second-rate existence, that's exactly what it will become. But if you
invest it with your interests, pleasures, and talents, this life-style can
be creative, fun, loving, and filled with accomplishment. It's not for
everybody, but it may be for you.

Growth and Change

As the wheel of the decade turns, so do a person's needs,
desires, and tasks. Each of us does, in effect, strike a
series of "deals," or compromises, between the wants and
needs of the inner self, and an outer environment that
offers certain possibilities and sets certain limitations. But
both the inner human being and the stability of outside
circumstances are always in a process of change.

— Maggie Scarf
From *Unfinished Business*[10]

Infertility has probably meant, for most of you, that life has stopped short. But, through grieving and ultimately resolving your grief, you may move on again.

Unfortunately, there is no way to cut short the grieving process—if you try, it will catch up with you sooner or later. You must struggle through the anger, sadness, and guilt in order to get to the other side. Grieving is letting go—letting go of unfulfilled dreams and replacing them with a comfortable reality.

People describe themselves in many ways after resolution— strong, calm, at peace, happy, self-assured. It is a time when the weight of the world feels lifted from their shoulders. I do not want to leave you with the impression, however, that infertility simply stops, for life, after infertility, is never the same. Whether the changes will be positive or negative depends on you.

Life has become more fragile and precious to me. I no longer take it for granted, at least not for long. There is a sense of appreciation for life that I think was always there but has now been strongly reawakened. It is like any crisis that happens to you instead of the other guy. It all of a sudden sharpens priorities and reminds you just what is important in life. We all forget at times, caught up in the hubbub of daily conflicts and disappointments, but memories of infertility set me straight.

My self-image and self-esteem have improved because I had to realize that I am a good, valuable person on my own. Having children won't make me any more worthy nor more whole. Having learned to cope with this problem has made me grow up and actually gives me a sense of pride and accomplishment. It's been a terrible struggle, but I'm getting through it.

Infertility has given me an acute appreciation of the child-parent relationship. All too often children are born to parents unexpectedly and become burdensome. Can you imagine being blind for thirteen years and then regaining your sight? How sweet would be the sights. The same goes for children born to a loving couple long childless. I know I'll be a better father from the experience.

The Aftermath of Infertility

Because infertility strikes with such intensity and causes so much change, you will feel its lingering effects for years to come. Most prominent is its effect on parenting. The appreciation for a child who has been so long in coming is enormous. Most parents feel great love for their children, but when parenthood follows a struggle with infertility, those feelings may be even more profound.

For the most part, such strong positive emotion is wonderful—your child will always know how much he was wanted and is loved. But it can also lead to some emotional traps you should watch out for. One common pitfall is overprotection of the child. Not allowing a child to grow independently, venture forth on his own when it is appropriate, and expand his skills at a normal pace can easily occur. Other two-year-olds might be climbing up the slide, but you may be too fearful of your child falling to let him do the same. Or you may feel that you must always be there at his side and refuse to allow even an occasional competent babysitter. Dealing with these fears is often helped by talking to and gaining support from other parents who share your anxieties.

Another common pitfall is an inability to become angry with or to discipline the child. If you do get angry and set limits, you may feel guilty for acting this way. Remember that you and the child are human like everyone else—there will be days when you have had it and days when the child is not the angel you fantasized about. Not only do you have a right to your feelings, but you should get angry at times. All children need discipline to give them direction and a sense of security as they grow toward independence. Spoiling that child you love so much will not be to his benefit.

Many find their feelings about having children have become so much stronger as the result of infertility that they change their minds about their role as parents. Many women, for example, who were very career-minded suddenly realize that their priorities have altered. They may decide that they no longer want to work, but instead want to be full-time mothers. There is no right or wrong way to handle this situation, but it is important for you to assess what your personal needs are.

Some men and women also feel guilty if they do not become the "perfect" parent. Having been through infertility, they need now to prove to others or themselves that they are capable of being the "best." This is, of course, an impossible expectation. Recognize that you will make mistakes and that you will have to learn the skills of parenting along the way like everybody else.

Going through infertility unquestionably provides an extraordinary appreciation for children that will probably never disappear. Even at the worst moments, you may be reminded of your Herculean efforts to have a family and why it was so important to you.

I now have two children, one adopted and one biological. They are two very pretty, very appealing little girls and I feel incredibly blessed. Infertility has caused me to cherish them, to never, ever take them for granted. When we are out and someone tells me how adorable they are, I think to myself, "You should only know how much I love them, how long they were in coming, how grateful I feel." Here is an example, although perhaps an odd one in some ways:

I recently took my four-year-old to have her hair cut at a fancy local hair salon. (I've since learned better!) She was impossible, crying and screaming and disrupting the whole salon. Then my eighteen-month-old, who was on my back, threw her orange juice all over the place. Other women, many of whom must have been mothers, glared at me without compassion. No one thought my children were adorable, and they looked at me with pity and scorn. For a moment, I was uncomfortable and embarrassed, tempted to run out the door and leave the little monsters behind. Then I thought to myself, "Remember the years of the thermometer; remember the anguish when your period arrived; remember how you felt different, left out, stuck in time." Then I realized—this is not a nightmare, it's a dream come true. This was what I wanted for so long!

I am ever aware that motherhood did not come naturally to me, and I really appreciate and enjoy the experience. I love the fact that people tell me how much

my older daughter looks like me and then ask where
my other one (the child I gave birth to) came from! I
love when others comment on how much my girls look
alike, not knowing they are of different genetic
backgrounds. I love the irony of it all, the surprise, the
fact that I am more contented than I ever was before.
My infertility was long and complicated, filled with
guilt and anger and confusion, but it has borne very
special fruit. I look back and I look around me with
disbelief and wonder.

Apart from the effects on parenting, the memories of infertility
can also linger on, often for many years, in a strange mixture of
sadness and joy. This does not necessarily mean that your infertility
remains unresolved. It only confirms how powerful the experience
has been and the depth of its impact.

It's been over a year since we adopted our son and two
years since the agonizing time when both my sister and
sister-in-law announced their pregnancies. Resolution
has come and, with it, tremendous changes in myself
and my life. Life has gone on. Friends have gotten
pregnant and had babies, but it hasn't produced the
same anguish in me that it did in years past. Pregnancy
isn't on my mind twenty-four hours a day, as it was at
that time. I'm casually aware of ovulation when it
occurs, but it doesn't carry the same emotional impact
and pressure to have sex. My cycles continue normally,
but I'm generally not aware of what day it is—that's a
nice feeling. Life is less frenetic, less structured, and
certainly more happy.

And then, yesterday, my sister-in-law announced
that she was pregnant again. I thought that I was
completely over the sadness and the pain, but there
were some of the same old feelings coming to haunt me
again. There wasn't the uncontrollable sobbing and the
sense that life was closing in on me. Just a lump in my
throat, a few tears, and a resurgence of wishes that it
could be me who was feeling life inside. But it wasn't.

I guess the lingering sadness will always have a

*small place inside me, regardless of the joys experienced
with my husband and son. I guess that I'll always
wonder what it's like to feel the movement of a child in
my belly or to first lay eyes on a baby that we have
produced—that perhaps has my husband's beautiful
hair or my small nose. I guess that's just the way life
is—you take the good and you take the bad, and you
make the best of what life dishes out. Maybe there will
come a time when the memories and sadness are
completely gone, but I doubt it. Perhaps what is
important is that I no longer feel that sense of total
emptiness inside because I've allowed my life to fill up
with joy in so many other ways. I just have to look in
my son's eyes and a surge of indescribable love and
fulfillment seems to flood within. That's what is so nice
about the human character—the capacity to ultimately
make the best out of whatever life provides. Infertility
has been the hardest experience in my life and will
linger on inside me, but it didn't destroy. In fact, I
grew—as a person, wife, friend, and eventually mother.*

It may be hard to believe now, but a time will come when you
are able to experience a powerful sense of accomplishment in conquering this crisis. By struggling, and growing through that struggle,
the ultimate rewards will be great. Having children has been much
harder for you than others, but, in the end, those efforts will bring a
sense of joy and satisfaction that is beyond compare.

Notes

Infertility: The Silent Struggle

1. Joseph H. Bellina, M.D., and Josleen Wilson, *You Can Have A Baby* (New York: Crown Publishers, 1985), xvi.

2. Ibid., 63.

3. Joseph H. Bellina, M.D., and Josleen Wilson, "Changing Fertility Risks," *Self,* April 1982.

4. Miriam Mazor, M.D., and Harriet F. Simons, *Infertility: Medical, Emotional, and Social Considerations* (New York: Human Sciences Press, 1984), xvii.

5. Robin Marantz Henig, "New Hope for Troubled Couples," *Woman's Day,* May 22, 1984, 40.

6. Bellina and Wilson, *You Can Have a Baby,* 79.

7. Otto Friedrich, "The New Origins of Life," *Time,* September 10, 1984, 50.

8. Ibid., 46.

9. Barbara Eck Menning, *Infertility: A Guide for the Childless Couple* (Englewood Cliffs, N.J.: Prentice-Hall, 1977), 6.

10. Diane Harris, "What It Costs to Fight Infertility," *Money,* December 1984, 202.

11. Henig, "New Hope for Troubled Couples," 43.

12. Matt Clark et al., "Infertility: New Cures, New Hopes," *Newsweek,* December 6, 1982, 102.

13. Harris, "What It Costs to Fight Infertility," 202.

14. Erik Erikson, *Childhood and Society* (New York: W.W. Norton and Co., 1950), 266–67.

15. Erma Bombeck, "Infertile Couples Should Come Out of the Closet," *Newsletter* (Northern New Jersey RESOLVE), April 1983, 2.

16. Ibid.

The Emotional Roller Coaster

1. Mary Beth Jorgensen, "On Healing," *Newsletter,* (New York City RESOLVE), July 1982, 3.

2. Emanuel Pariser, "A Man's Point of View," *Newsletter* (RESOLVE), April 1985, 3.

3. Ibid.

4. Mazor and Simons, eds., *Infertility,* 23.

5. Machelle M. Seibel, M.D., and Melvin L. Taymor, M.D., "Emotional Aspects of Infertility," *Fertility and Sterility* 37 (February 1982): 137.

6. Herman C. B. Denber, "Psychiatric Aspects of Infertility," *Journal of Reproductive Medicine* 20 (January 1978): 28.

7. Seibel and Taymor, "Emotional Aspects of Infertility," 144.

8. John J. Stangel, M.D., *Fertility and Conception: An Essential Guide for Childless Couples* (New York: Paddington Press, 1979), 86–87.

Infertile in a Fertile Society

1. Excerpt from letter published in *Perspectives on Infertility*, November-December 1982, 5.

Infertility and the Couple

1. Aaron L. Rutledge, "Husband-Wife Conferences in the Home," in *Handbook of Marriage Counseling*, ed. Ben N. Ard, Jr., and Constance C. Ard (Palo Alto, Calif.: Science and Behavior Books, 1969), 344.

2. Merle Bombardieri, "The Twenty-Minute Rule: First-Aid for Couples in Distress," *Newsletter* (RESOLVE), December 1983, 5.

3. Israel W. Charny, *Marital Love and Hate* (New York: Macmillan Company, 1972), 122.

4. James Leslie McCary, *Freedom and Growth in Marriage* (Santa Barbara, Calif.: Hamilton Publishing Co., 1975), 275.

5. Ibid., 270.

6. John Williams, "Feedback Techniques in Marriage Counseling," in *Handbook of Marriage Counseling*, ed. Ard and Ard, 349.

Infertility and Sex

1. Menning, *Infertility*, 129.

2. Bellina and Wilson, *You Can Have a Baby*, 302.

3. Deidre Laiken, "Impotence—What Causes It and What Both of You Can Do to Help," *Glamour*, September 1984, 138.

4. James Leslie McCary, *Human Sexuality* (New York: D. Van Nostrand Co., 1973), 163.

5. AMA Committee on Human Sexuality, *Human Sexuality* (N.p. American Medical Association, 1972), 114.

6. Ibid., 115.

7. McCary, *Freedom and Growth in Marriage*, 218.

8. Lonnie Barbach, *For Each Other* (Garden City, N.Y.: Anchor Press/Doubleday, 1982), 232.

9. Ibid., 267.

10. Menning, *Infertility*, 131.

Surviving the Infertility Grind

1. *Newsletter* (RESOLVE), June 1982, 7.

2. Herbert Benson, M.D., *The Relaxation Response* (New York: William Morrow & Co., 1975), 114–15.

3. Edward A. Charlesworth and Ronald G. Nathan, *Stress Management* (New York: Atheneum, 1984), 50–51.

4. Ibid., 65–67.

5. David A. Feigley, "Psychological Burnout in High-Level Athletes," *Physician and Sportsmedicine* 12 (October 1984), 110.

6. Frederic Leer, "Running as an Adjunct to Psychotherapy," *Social Work* 25 (January 1980): 21.

7. Stangel, *Fertility and Conception*, 158–159.

8. Menning, *Infertility*, 160.

Infertility and Religion

1. Sharon Buttry, "Infertility: A Spiritual Journey," *Newsletter* (RESOLVE), December 1982, 5.

2. Judith Stigger, *Coping with Infertility* (Minneapolis: Augsburg Publishing House, 1983), 91–95.

3. Harold S. Kushner, *When Bad Things Happen to Good People* (New York: Avon Book, 1981), 10.

4. Stigger, *Coping with Infertility*, 89.

5. Susan Miller, "Family Bible Study," *Stepping Stones*, June 1985, 4.

6. Kushner, *When Bad Things Happen to Good People*, 125.

7. Blu Greenberg, *How to Run a Traditional Jewish Household* (New York: Simon & Schuster, 1983), 122.

8. Marsha Sheinfeld, "Infertility and Orthodox Judaism," *Newsletter* (RESOLVE), June 1982, 5.

9. Chris Probst, "Religion and Infertility—Feelings from an Infertile Mormon," *Newsletter* (RESOLVE), January 1982, 5.

10. Lori Andrews, *New Conceptions: A Consumer Guide to the Newest Infertility Treatments* (New York: St. Martin's Press, 1984), 187–88.

The Doctor-Patient Relationship

1. Marvin S. Belsky, M.D., and Leonard Gross, *How to Choose and Use Your Doctor* (New York: Arbor House, 1975).

Issues of Special Concern

1. Robin Marantz Henig, "New Hope for Troubled Couples," *Woman's Day*, May 22, 1984, 43.

2. Menning, *Infertility*, 137.

3. McCary, *Freedom and Growth in Marriage*, 295–96.

4. Cecile Terrien Lampton, *Newsletter* (New York City RESOLVE), May 1982, 4.

5. "The Emotional Impact of Miscarriage," *Special Publication*, RESOLVE, 1980, 1.

6. Hank Pizer and Christine O'Brien, *Coping with a Miscarriage* (New York: Dial Press, 1980), 15.

7. Ibid., 13.

8. Menning, *Infertility*, 70.

9. Tim Page, "Life Miscarried," *New York Times Magazine*, January 27, 1985, 50.

10. Elisabeth Herz, M.D., "Psychological Repercussions of Pregnancy Loss," *Psychiatric Annals* 14 (June 1984): 454.

11. Harry C. Huneycutt, M.D., and Judith L. Davis, *All about Hysterectomy* (New York: Reader's Digest Press, 1977), 278.

12. William H. Masters and Virginia E. Johnson, "Endometriosis, Surgery, and Hysterectomy," *Special Publication*, The Endometriosis Association, Inc., 1983, 2.

13. Ibid., 261.

14. Merle J. Berger and Donald P. Goldstein, "Infertility Related to Exposure to DES in Utero," in *Infertility*, ed. Mazor and Simons, 158.

15. Roberta J. Apfel and Susan M. Fisher, "Emotional Aspects of DES Exposure," in *Infertility*, ed. Mazor and Simons, 177.

16. Alan B. Retik and Stuart B. Bauer, "Infertility Related to DES Exposure in Utero: Reproductive Problems in the Male," in *Infertility*, Mazor and Simons, 170–71.

17. Apfel and Fisher, "Emotional Aspects of DES Exposure," 173.

The High Technology of Parenthood

1. "Emotional Aspects of AID," *Newsletter* (New York City RESOLVE) February 1984, 4.

2. Bellina and Wilson, *You Can Have a Baby*, 313.

3. Andrews, *New Conceptions*, 178.

4. Silber, *How to Get Pregnant*, 175.

5. Barbara Eck Menning, "Psychosocial Issues in Artificial Insemination by Donor," *Newsletter* (RESOLVE), April 1980, 5.

6. Ibid.

7. David M. Berger, M.D., "Psychological Aspects of Donor Insemination," *International Journal of Psychiatry in Medicine* 12 (January 1982): 54.

8. Anne Fadiman, "Small Miracles of Love and Science," *Life*, November 1982, 50.

9. Michael Kramer, "Last-Chance Babies," *New York*, August 12, 1985, 37.

10. M. R. Soules, "The In Vitro Fertilization Pregnancy Rate: "Let's Be Honest with One Another," *Fertility and Sterility* 43 (April 1985): 511.

11. Otto Friedrich, "The New Origins of Life," *Time*, September 10, 1984, 48.

12. Andrews, *New Conceptions*, 123.

13. Charles Wilkes, M.D., et al., "Pregnancy Related to Infertility Diagnosis, Number of Attempts, and Age in a Program of In Vitro Fertilization," *Obstetrics and Gynecology* 66 (September 1985): 350.

14. Andrews, *New Conceptions*, 139.

15. "Fertility Rights—Medical Efforts to Help Childless Couples Pose Host of Difficult Issues," *Wall Street Journal* 204, no. 26:14.

16. Friedrich, "The New Origins of Life," 55.

17. Ibid., 54.

18. "Surrogates: Alternative to Adoption," *Kansas City Star*, May 23, 1982, 1A.

19. "Surrogate Mothers, Couples Charting New Territory," *Wichita Eagle-Beacon*, August 21, 1983, 8A.

20. Andrews, *New Conceptions*, 228.

The Crossroads of Infertility

1. Miriam Mazor, M.D., "Barren Couples," *Psychology Today* 12 (May 1979), 108.

2. "On Healing," *Newsletter* (New York City RESOLVE), July 1982.

3. Menning, *Infertility*, 115.

4. McCary, *Freedom and Growth in Marriage*, 317.

Ending the Struggle

1. "Adoption: Myth vs. Fact," *Perspectives on Infertility*, May-June 1983, 13.

2. Ibid.

3. Edmund Blair Bolles, *The Penguin Adoption Handbook* (New York: Penguin Books, 1984), 28.

4. Mary Kuntz, "Paying Expenses Is Legal, Buying Babies Is Not," *Forbes*, December 31, 1984, 128.

5. *Newsletter* (RESOLVE), September 1984, 2.

6. Merle Bombardieri, "Childfree Decision-Making," Special Publication, RESOLVE, 3.

7. Anne Smith, "Childfree Living," *Newsletter* (New York City RESOLVE), July 1985, 8.

8. Bombardieri, "Childfree Decision-Making," 3.

9. Ibid., 9.

10. Maggie Scarf, *Unfinished Business: Pressure Points in the Lives of Women* (Garden City, N.Y.: Doubleday, 1980).

Bibliography

General

AMELAR, RICHARD D., M.D.; DUBIN, LAWRENCE, M.D.; AND WALSH, PATRICK C., M.D. *Male Infertility*. Philadelphia: W. B. Saunders Co., 1977.

BEANS, BRUCE E. "Beating Infertility." *Philadelphia*, September 1985, 127–31.

BELLINA, JOSEPH H., M.D., AND WILSON, JOSLEEN. "Changing Fertility Risks." *Self*, April 1982.

BELLINA, JOSEPH H., M.D., AND WILSON, JOSLEEN. *You Can Have a Baby*. New York: Crown Publishers, 1985.

BERNSTEIN, JUDITH, AND MATTOX, JOHN H., M.D. "An Overview of Infertility." *JOGN Nursing*, September-October 1982, 309–14.

BOSTON WOMEN'S HEALTH BOOK COLLECTIVE. *Our Bodies, Ourselves*. New York: Simon & Schuster, 1985.

COMAN, CAROLYN. "Trying (and Trying and Trying) to Get Pregnant." *Ms.*, May 1983, 21–24.

CORSON, STEPHEN L., M.D. *Conquering Infertility*. Norwalk, Conn.: Appleton-Century-Crofts, 1983.

GARCIA, CEISO-RAMON, M.D.; MASTROIANNI, LUIGI, M.D.; AMELAR, RICHARD, M.D.; AND DUBIN, LAWRENCE, M.D., eds. *Current Therapy of Infertility, 1984-1985*. Philadelphia: B. C. Decker, 1984.

GRIMES, ELWYN M. "For Infertile Couples—A Holistic Approach." *Contemporary OB/GYN*, February 1984, 179-.

HARRISON, MARY. *Infertility: A Guide for Couples*. Boston: Houghton Mifflin Co., 1977.

MAZOR, MIRIAM D., M.D., AND SIMONS, HARRIET F., eds. *Infertility: Medical, Emotional, and Social Considerations*. New York: Human Sciences Press, 1984.

MENNING, BARBARA ECK. *Infertility: A Guide for the Childless Couple*. Englewood Cliffs, N.J.: Prentice-Hall, 1977.

MOGHISSI, KAMRAN S., M.D., AND WALLACH, EDWARD E., M.D. "Unexplained Infertility." *Fertility and Sterility* 39 (January 1983): 5.

MOSHER, WILLIAM D., AND PRATT, WILLIAM F. "Fecundity and Infertility in the United States, 1965-82." Arlington, Va.: National Center for Health Statistics, 1985.

OLDER, JULIA. *Endometriosis*. New York: Charles Scribner's Sons, 1984.

SILBER, SHERMAN J., M.D. *How to Get Pregnant*. New York: Charles Scribner's Sons, 1980.

STANGEL, JOHN J., M.D. *Fertility and Conception: An Essential Guide for Childless Couples*. New York: Paddington Press, 1979.

ZIMMERMAN, DAVID R. "The Shocking Reason More and More Young Women Can't Have Babies." *Good Housekeeping*, March 1985, 26–33.

284

Social-Emotional Aspects of Infertility

BOMBARDIERI, MERLE. "Coping with the Stress of Infertility." Special Publication from RESOLVE.

DENBER, HERMAN C. B., M.D. "Psychiatric Aspects of Infertility." *Journal of Reproductive Medicine* 20 (January 1978):23–29.

HALVERSON, KAYE, AND HESS, KAREN M. *The Wedded Unmother*. Minneapolis, Minn.: Augsburg Publishing House, 1980.

HARRIS, DIANE. "What It Costs to Fight Infertility." *Money*, December 1984, 201–12.

HINTON, MARGARET. "The Stress of Infertility—and How to Cope!" Special Publication of Minnesota RESOLVE.

JOHNSTON, PATRICIA IRWIN. *Understanding: A Guide to Impaired Fertility for Family and Friends*. Fort Wayne, Ind.: Perspectives Press, 1983.

LEADER, ARTHUR, M.D.; TAYLOR, PATRICK J., M.D.; AND DANILUK, JUDITH. "Infertility: Clinical and Psychological Aspects." *Psychiatric Annals* 14 (June 1984): 461–67.

MAZOR, MIRIAM, M.D. "Barren Couples." *Psychology Today* 12 (May 1979):101–12.

MAZOR, MIRIAM D., M.D. "Psychosexual Problems of the Infertile Couple." *Medical Aspects of Human Sexuality* 14 (December 1980):32–49.

McGUIRE, LINDA S. "Psychologic Management of Infertile Women." *Postgraduate Medicine* 57 (May 1975):173–76.

MENNING, BARBARA ECK. "Counseling Infertile Couples." *Contemporary OB/GYN* 13 (February 1979):101–8.

MENNING, BARBARA ECK. "The Emotional Needs of Infertile Couples." *Fertility and Sterility* 34 (October 1980):313–19.

MITCHARD, JACQUELYN. *Mother Less Child*. New York: W.W. Norton & Co., 1985.

ROSENFELD, DAVID L., M.D., and MITCHELL, EILEEN. "Treating the Emotional Aspects of Infertility: Counseling Services in an Infertility Clinic." *American Journal of Obstetrics and Gynecology* 135 (September 15, 1979):177–80.

SEIBEL, MACHELLE M., M.D., AND TAYMOR, MELVIN L., M.D. "Emotional Aspects of Infertility." *Fertility and Sterility* 37 (February 1982):137–45.

SHREDNICK, ANDREA. "The Emotional Outlet—Male Sexual Dysfunction." *Perspectives on Infertility* 1 (May-June 1983):15–16.

STAMELL, MARCIA. "Infertility: Fighting Back." *New York*, March 21, 1983, 32–40.

STIGGER, JUDITH A. *Coping with Infertility*. Minneapolis, Minn.: Augsburg Publishing House, 1983.

Sexual Issues

BARBACH, LONNIE. *For Each Other: Sharing Sexual Intimacy*. Garden City, N.Y.: Anchor Press/Doubleday, 1982.

BARBACH, LONNIE. *For Yourself: The Fulfillment of Female Sexuality*. Garden City, N.Y.: Anchor Press/Doubleday, 1975.

COMFORT, ALEX, ed. *The Joy of Sex*. New York: Simon & Schuster, 1972.

FLEMING, JOHN L., M.D. "Occasional Impotence." *Medical Aspects of Human Sexuality* 19 (July 1985):52–66.

GELINAS, PAUL J. *Coping with Sexual Problems*. New York: Richards Rosen Press, 1981.

LAIKEN, DEIRDRE. "Impotence—What Causes It and What Both of You Can Do to Help." *Glamour*, September 1984, 138-.

MASTERS, WILLIAM H., and JOHNSON, VIRGINIA. *The Pleasure Principle*. Boston: Little, Brown & Co., 1974.

PENNEY, ALEXANDRA. *How to Make Love to a Man*. New York: Clarkson N. Potter, 1981.

PENNEY, ALEXANDRA. *How to Make Love to Each Other.* New York: G. P. Putnam's, 1982.

PENNEY, ALEXANDRA. *Great Sex.* New York: G. P. Putnam's, 1985.

PHILLIPS, DEBORA. *Sexual Confidence.* Boston: Houghton Mifflin, 1980.

Doctor-Patient Relationship

BELSKY, MARVIN S., M.D., AND GROSS, LEONARD. *How to Choose and Use Your Doctor.* New York: Arbor House, 1975.

BLUESTONE, NAOMI, M.D. "What's up Doc?" *Health,* March 1985, 76.

Pregnancy Loss

BEREZIN, NANCY. *After a Loss in Pregnancy.* New York: Simon & Schuster, 1982.

BORG, SUSAN, AND LASKER, JUDITH. *When Pregnancy Fails.* Boston: Beacon Press, 1981.

FRIEDMAN, ROCHELLE, M.D., AND GRADSTEIN, BONNIE. *Surviving Pregnancy Loss.* Boston: Little, Brown & Co., 1982.

HERZ, ELISABETH, M.D. "Psychological Repercussions of Pregnancy Loss." *Psychiatric Annals* 14 (June 1984):454–57.

PIZER, HANK, AND O'BRIEN, CHRISTINE. *Coping with a Miscarriage.* New York: Dial Press, 1980.

Hysterectomy

GIUSTINI, F.G., M.D., AND KEEFER, F.J., M.D. *Understanding Hysterectomy.* New York: Walker & Co., 1979.

HUNEYCUTT, HARRY C., M.D., AND DAVIS, JUDITH L. *All about Hysterectomy.* New York: Reader's Digest Press, 1977.

MORGAN, SUSANNE. *Coping with a Hysterectomy.* New York: Dial Press, 1982.

DES Exposure

BICHLER, JOYCE. *DES Daughter: A True Story of Tragedy and Triumph.* New York: Avon Books, 1981.

CLAPP, DIANE. "DES: Its Impact on Infertility." Special Publication from RESOLVE.

ORENBERG, CYNTHIA LAITMAN. *DES: The Complete Story.* New York: St. Martin's Press, 1981.

SCHWARTZ, RUTH W., M.D., AND STEWART, NANCY B. "Psychological Effects of Diethylstilbestrol Exposure." *Journal of the American Medical Association* 237 (January 17, 1977):252–54.

STILLMAN, R. J. "Pregnancy Prospects of DES Daughters." *Contemporary OB/GYN* 24 (October 1984):47–53.

TURIEL, JUDITH. "The Doctors I Can't Forgive." *Redbook,* February 1981, 44–50.

The High Technology of Parenthood

ALSOFROM, JUDY. "The New Sexual Revolution—Human Reproduction." *Self,* December 1984, 64–68.

ANDREWS, LORI. *New Conceptions: A Consumer Guide to the Newest Infertility Treatments.* New York: St. Martin's Press, 1984.

BECK, WILLIAM W., M.D., AND WALLACH, EDWARD E., M.D. "When Therapy Fails—Artificial Insemination." *Contemporary OB/GYN* 17 (January 1981):113–25.

BELLINA, JOSEPH H., M.D., AND WILSON, JOSLEEN. "How to Have a Test Tube Baby." *Glamour,* May 1985, 122–33.

BOMBARDIERI, MERLE, AND CLAPP, DIANE. "Reducing the Stress of In Vitro Fertilization." *Contemporary OB/GYN* 24 (October 1984):91–99.

CLAPP, DIANE. "In Vitro Fertilization: An Overview." Special Publication from RESOLVE.

CLARK, MATT, ET AL. "Infertility: New Cures, New Hopes." *Newsweek*, December 6, 1982, 102–10.

DAVID, AMNON, M.D., AND AVIDAN, DALIA. "Artificial Insemination Donor: Clinical and Psychologic Aspects." *Fertility and Sterility* 27 (May 1976):528–32.

FADIMAN, ANNE. "Small Miracles of Love and Science." *Life*, November 1982, 44–52.

FRIEDRICH, OTTO. "The New Origins of Life," *Time*, September 10, 1984, 46–56.

GORNEY, CYNTHIA. "The Other Mothers." *California*, October 1983.

HANDEL, WILLIAM W., AND SHERWYN, BERNARD A. "Surrogate Parenting." *Trial* 18 (April 1982):57–60.

HARVEY, BARBARA, AND HARVEY, ALLEN. "How Couples Feel about Donor Insemination." *Contemporary OB/GYN* 9 (June 1977):93–97.

HENIG, ROBIN MARANTZ. "New Hope for Troubled Couples." *Woman's Day*, May 22, 1984, 32–43.

JOHNSTON, IAN; LOPATA, ALEX; SPEIRS, ANDREW; HOULT, IAN; KELLOW, GEOFF; AND DU PLESSIS, YVONNE. "In Vitro Fertilization: The Challenge of the Eighties." *Fertility and Sterility* 36 (December 1981):699–706.

KEANE, NOEL P., AND BREO, DENNIS L. *The Surrogate Mother*. New York: Everest House, 1981.

KRAMER, MICHAEL. "Last-Chance Babies." *New York*, August 12, 1985, 34–42.

MACHOL, LIBBY. "Referring Your Patient for In Vitro Fertilization." *Contemporary OB/GYN* 23 (January 1984):127–42.

MENNING, BARBARA ECK. "Psychosocial Issues in Artificial Insemination by Donor." Special Publication from RESOLVE.

THOMPSON, W., AND BOYLE, D. D. "Counseling Patients for Artificial Insemination and Subsequent Pregnancy." *Clinics in Obstetrics and Gynaecology* 9 (April 1982):211–23.

WALTZER, HERBERT, M.D. "Psychological and Legal Aspects of Artificial Insemination (A.I.D.): An Overview." *American Journal of Psychotherapy* 36 (January 1982):91–102.

WILKES, CHARLES A., M.D.; ROSENWAKS, ZEV, M.D.; JONES, DEBRA L., and JONES, HOWARD W., JR., M.D. "Pregnancy Related to Infertility Diagnosis, Number of Attempts, and Age in a Program of In Vitro Fertilization." *Obstetrics and Gynecology* 66 (September 1985):350–52.

Adoption

ARMS, SUZANNE. *To Love and Let Go*. New York: Knopf, 1983.

BOLLES, EDMUND BLAIR. *The Penguin Adoption Handbook*. New York: Penguin Books, 1984.

BRINLEY, MARYANN BUCKNAM. "The Baby Business." *McCalls*, June 1985, 89–.

BUNIN, SHERRY. "If You're Planning to Adopt: Essential Reading." *Parents*, March 1985, 42–48.

BURGESS, LINDA CANNON. *The Art of Adoption*. New York: W. W. Norton, 1976.

DYWASUK, COLETTE TAUBE. *Adoption—Is It for You?* New York: Harper & Row, 1973.

GILMAN, LOIS. *The Adoption Resource Book*. New York: Harper & Row, 1984.

GRADSTEIN, BONNIE; GRADSTEIN, MARK; AND GLASS, ROBERT. "Private Adoption." *Fertility and Sterility* 37 (April 1982):548–52.

HALLENBECK, CAROL A. *Our Child: Preparation for Parenting in Adoption—Instructor's Guide*. Wayne, Pa.: Our Child Press, 1984.

JOHNSTON, PATRICIA IRWIN. *An Adopter's Advocate*. Fort Wayne, Ind: Perspectives Press, 1984.

JOHNSTON, PATRICIA IRWIN, ed. *Perspectives on a Grafted Tree*. Fort Wayne, Ind.: Perspectives Press, 1984.

LOVENHEIM, BARBARA. "The Baby Brokers." *Redbook*, October 1983, 102-.

KREMENTZ, JILL. *How It Feels to Be Adopted*. New York: Knopf, 1982.

KUNTZ, MARY. "Paying Expenses Is Legal, Buying Babies Is Not." *Forbes*, December, 31, 1984, 128–30.

MACHOL, LIBBY. "Report on Adoption, 1982." *Contemporary OB/GYN* 19 (February 1982):65-.

MANKITA, BEN. "The Crossroads of Infertility: Moving towards Adoption." *Perspectives on Infertility* 1 (May-June 1983):5–15.

MARTIN, CYNTHIA. *Beating the Adoption Game*. La Jolla, Calif.: Oak Tree Publications, 1980.

MCNAMARA, JOAN. *The Adoption Advisor*. New York: Hawthorn Books, 1975.

PLUMEZ, JACQUELINE HORNOR. *Successful Adoption*. New York: Harmony Books, 1982.

RENNE, DIANE. "'There's Always Adoption': The Infertility Problem." *Child Welfare* 56 (July 1977):465–70.

SMITH, JEROME, AND MIROF, FRANKLIN I. *You're Our Child*. Washington, D.C.: University Press of America, 1981.

Childfree Living

BOMBARDIERI, MERLE. *The Baby Decision*. New York: Rawson, Wade Publishers, 1981.

BOMBARDIERI, MERLE. "Childfree Decision-Making." Special Publication from RESOLVE.

BURGWYN, DIANA. *Marriage without Children*. New York: Harper & Row, 1981.

FABE, MARILYN, AND WIKLER, NORMA. *Up against the Clock: Career Women Speak on the Choice to Have Children*. New York: Random House, 1979.

LINDSAY, KAREN. *Friends as Family*. Boston: Beacon Press, 1981.

WHELAN, ELIZABETH. *A Baby? . . . Maybe*. New York: Bobbs-Merrill, 1975.

Related Books and Articles to Help with Coping

BENSON, HERBERT, M.D. *The Relaxation Response*. New York: William Morrow & Co., 1975.

BRODERICK, CARLFRED. *Couples—How to Confront Problems and Maintain Loving Relationships*. New York: Simon & Schuster, 1979.

CARRINGTON, PATRICIA. *Releasing: The New Behavioral Science Method for Dealing with Pressure Situations*. New York: William Morrow, 1984.

CHARLESWORTH, EDWARD A., AND NATHAN, RONALD G. *Stress Management*. New York: Atheneum, 1984.

KAPPELMAN, MURRAY, M.D. *Raising the Only Child*. New York: E. P. Dutton, 1975.

KUBLER-ROSS, ELISABETH. *On Death and Dying*. New York: Macmillan Co., 1969.

KUSHNER, HAROLD S. *When Bad Things Happen to Good People*. New York: Avon Books, 1981.

LASSWELL, MARCIA, AND LOBSENZ, NORMAN M. *No-Fault Marriage*. New York: Ballantine Books, 1976.

MCCARY, JAMES LESLIE. *Freedom and Growth in Marriage*. Santa Barbara, Calif.: Hamilton Publishing Co., 1975.

SCHWARTZ, JACKIE. *Letting Go of Stress*. New York: Pinnacle, 1982.

STEARNS, ANN KAISER. *Living through Personal Crisis*. New York: Ballantine Books, 1985.

TATELBAUM, JUDY. *The Courage to Grieve*. New York: Harper & Row, 1980.

Periodicals and Newsletters on Infertility

Fertility News, North Duke Professional Center, 4020 North Roxboro Road,

Durham, NC 27704. (Bimonthly medical source for the infertile couple/consumer.)

Loving Arms, Pregnancy and Infant Loss Center of Minnesota, 1415 E. Wayzota Boulevard, Suite 22, Wayzota, MN 55391.

Perspectives on Infertility, Center for Communications in Infertility, P.O. Box 516, Yorktown Heights, NY 10598.

RESOLVE *Newsletter*, Resolve, Inc., P.O. Box 474, Belmont, MA 02178. (Resolve, Inc. also has an infertility bibliography that is continually updated.)

Stepping Stones, P.O. Box 11141, Wichita, KN 67211 (Free bimonthly newsletter for Christian infertile couples).

Resources

Infertility Organizations and Support Groups

RESOLVE, Inc., P.O. Box 474, Belmont, MA 02178 (617/484-2424).
A national nonprofit organization for infertile individuals and
couples. There are over forty chapters throughout the United
States. Services include telephone counseling, referral to
medical and related services, support groups, and public
education through newsletters, fact sheets, and chapter
meetings.

American Fertility Society, 2131 Magnolia Avenue, Birmingham, AL
35256.
The national organization for infertility specialists. It will
provide you with medical referrals by listing member
physicians in your area but will not give recommendations. It
also publishes the medical journal *Fertility and Sterility.*

The Barren Foundation, 230 North Michigan St., Chicago, IL
60601.
An organization dedicated to research and public education in
the field of reproductive endocrinology. Services include
support groups, medical seminars, and literature on infertility.

Center for Communications in Infertility, Inc., P.O. Box 516,
Yorktown Heights, NY 10598.
Publishes the bimonthly magazine, *Perspectives on Infertility*,
which covers both medical and emotional aspects of
infertility.

American College of Obstetricians and Gynecologists, 600
Maryland Ave., S.W., Suite 300 East, Washington, DC 20024.

An organization of board-certified obstetricians and gynecologists. It will provide you with the names of infertility specialists in your area but will not give recommendations.

Endometriosis

Endometriosis Association, P.O. Box 92187, Milwaukee, WI 53202.
A self-help organization for women with endometriosis and others who are interested in exchanging information about the disease. Services include crisis call help, local chapters and support groups, a national newsletter, fact sheets and brochures, and educational programs. A data registry of individuals' experiences with endometriosis is also available to members and researchers.

Adoption Organizations (Providing Information and Support)

The Open Door Society of Massachusetts, Inc., 867 Boylston St., Boston, MA 02116.
A volunteer, nonprofit organization of adoptive, foster, and prospective parents; concerned professionals; and interested others. It is not an adoption agency but helps to find permanent families for special needs children. It also offers support to families before, during, and after placement. *ODS News* is published bimonthly.

OURS, Inc. (Organization for a United Response), 3307 Highway 100 North, Suite 203, Minneapolis, MN 55422.
A private, nonprofit support organization for adoptive and prospective adoptive families, as well as interested professionals. It is especially concerned with the adoption of foreign born and special needs children. Services include *OURS* magazine (published bimonthly), updated listings of agencies and information on adoption, Helpline (a family-to-family support system), and the sale of books and special merchandise for adoptive families. There are over one hundred chapters throughout the United States.

Families Adopting Children Everywhere (F.A.C.E.), P.O. Box 28058, Northwood Station, Baltimore, MD 21239.
An adoptive-parent support group whose goal is to help

people adopt children from the United States and foreign countries. Services include information and support to prospective parents, a six-week course entitled "Family Building through Adoption," bimonthly public meetings, a monthly newsletter, social events, and help in adopting "waiting" children.

The Latin America Parents Association, P.O. Box 72, Seaford, NY 11783.

A nonprofit, volunteer organization whose goal is to help those seeking to adopt children from Latin America. Services include information about adoption and naturalization requirements, fact sheets, informational meetings, cultural and social events, and a bimonthly newsletter.

National Committee for Adoption (NCFA), Suite 326, 1346 Connecticut Ave., N.W., Washington, DC 20036.

An organization that supports agency adoption. It provides information about adoption and infertility, works for sound standards of professional practice, looks into the impact of current adoption practices, and develops and works with state committees for adoption. A variety of publications are available through NCFA.

North American Council on Adoptable Children (NACAC), 810 18th St. N.W., Suite 703, Washington, DC 20006.

A national organization that coordinates over six hundred adoption support/advocacy groups in the United States and Canada. It can help you find a parents group in your area, as well as provide you with general information on adoption. It has a monthly publication, ADOPTALK.

National Adoption Exchange, 1218 Chestnut St., Philadelphia, PA 19107.

An organization helping to find permanent families for special needs children. Families that have already completed home studies can register with the exchange, which will then try to match children with families. A newsletter and photolisting book are available through the organization.

International Concerns Committee for Children, 911 Cypress Dr., Boulder, CO 80303.

Publishes the *Report on Foreign Adoption*, a directory of the latest intercountry adoption information (including agencies and agents, countries where babies are available, waiting times, costs, and laws).

Parents for Private Adoption, P.O. Box 7, Pawlet, VT 05761.
A support and education group for prospective and adoptive families, birthparents, adoptees, relatives, professionals, and other concerned individuals. Present and planned services include a lengthy newsletter, educational and supportive meetings, adoption literature, workshops, networking, research, and a resume service.

The Penguin Adoption Handbook offers a state-by-state directory of adoptive parent organizations.

The Adoption Resource Book offers a state-by-state directory of domestic and intercountry adoption agencies.

INDEX